The MALE BIOLOGICAL CLOCK

THE STARTLING NEWS ABOUT AGING, SEXUALITY, AND FERTILITY IN MEN

Harry Fisch, M.D.
with Stephen Braun

FREE PRESS

New York   London   Toronto   Sydney

*f*P

FREE PRESS
A Division of Simon & Schuster, Inc.
1230 Avenue of the Americas
New York, NY 10020

FREE PRESS and colophon are trademarks of Simon & Schuster, Inc.

For information about special discounts for bulk purchases,
please contact Simon & Schuster Special Sales:
1-800-456-6798 or business@simonandschuster.com

Designed by Dana Sloan
Interior illustrations by Nancy Heim

Manufactured in the United States of America

1   3   5   7   9   10   8   6   4   2

Library of Congress Cataloging-in-Publication Data
Fisch, Harry.
The male biological clock : the startling news about aging, sexuality,
and fertility in men / Harry Fisch with Stephen Braun.
p.   cm.
Includes index.
1. Infertility, Male. 2. Generative organs, Male—Aging. I. Braun, Stephen. II. Title.
RC889.F49 2005   616.6'92—dc22   2004057701

ISBN 0-7432-5991-2

To whom I am most devoted, my wife, Karen;
and our children—David, Melissa, and Sam.

Contents

The

MALE
BIOLOGICAL
CLOCK

INTRODUCTION

The Silent Epidemic

Say "biological clock," and most people think "women." Most people know that a woman's ovaries stop producing eggs at some point and that natural fertility ends with menopause. But conventional wisdom holds that men can father children as easily at seventy-five as at twenty-five. Stories of people such as Saul Bellow, who became a father at age eighty-five, and Tony Randall, a father at seventy-two, help sustain a widespread myth: women have a gun to their heads that men never have to face.

Unfortunately, the conventional wisdom is wrong. Men have biological clocks too. This fundamental fact about life has been very slow to reach the public for many reasons, not least because an entire industry has arisen in the past decade for "fixing" *female* infertility with high-tech procedures such as *in vitro* fertilization (IVF). By and large, treating female infertility is much more financially lucrative than treating male infertility. The focus (by both women and their doctors) on the female side of infertility, and the urgency with which many couples come to the fertility industry, combine to shove male infertility to the sidelines and to launch couples into IVF prematurely. Sadly, millions of dollars are spent each year on IVF and other sophisticated procedures that could have been avoided if the male side of infertility had been properly diagnosed and treated. Most people—and even many doctors—don't know the startling facts about aging, male sexuality, and male infertility, in part because the studies that reveal these facts are so new.

The male biological clock isn't like a woman's. It "ticks" at a different rate, it causes an entirely different set of bodily and behavioral changes over the course of a lifetime, and it doesn't strike a "midnight" toll of an absolute end to fertility. But male fertility, testosterone levels, and sexuality all definitely decline with age. Men older than thirty-five are twice as likely to be infertile as men twenty-five or younger.[1,2] In addition, as men age, the genetic quality of their sperm declines significantly.[3] Every couple should know these facts because they affect two of the most important things in their life: their ability to have children and their capacity to have good sex.

The reality of the male biological clock and the ways the ticking of this clock can result in numerous problems with fertility or sexuality are facts that have not yet reached the men and women on the street. On the contrary: myths about male infertility and sexuality abound. Here are the myths I come across most often.

1. *Infertility is rare and is mostly a women's problem.*

   Wrong. Each year about 6 million American men and women realize they have a fertility problem. In about 40 percent of these couples the problem lies with the man. In another 40 percent, it's the woman with the problem, and in another 20 percent either both partners contribute or the cause is unknown. Roughly 10 percent of men trying to father a child—roughly 2.5 million men in the United States alone—are either infertile or subfertile. Many of these men don't know they have a problem because they haven't been tested; others have been tested but not thoroughly enough. Hence their problem remains undetected and medical attention shifts to the female.

2. *Although older women are at higher risk of having children with Down syndrome, the man's age doesn't matter.*

   Wrong. Down syndrome is a pattern of mental retardation and altered physical features caused by an extra chromosome 21. It has long been known that a woman's chance of having a baby with Down syndrome rises dramatically after age thirty-five, but it had been thought that the man's age had nothing to do with it. Now we know that this is false—men also have a higher likelihood of fathering a Down syndrome baby as they get older. The incidence of genetic problems in their sperm increases with age, which leads to many problems, including Down syndrome. In fact, a recent study found that half the cases of Down syndrome in children born to women older than thirty-five are likely to be sperm-related.[4]

3. *Men with no sperm in their semen are sterile.*

Wrong. In the past, this statement was true, but today numerous methods exist for extracting sperm from the testicles or other parts of the male reproductive tract and using the harvested sperm to fertilize a woman's eggs, using advanced reproductive technologies.

4. *A vasectomy is final; it cannot be reversed.*

Wrong. In fact, every year roughly 5,000 men with vasectomies change their minds, and today, with the advent of microsurgical techniques, the success rate for vasectomy reversal in the hands of a competent surgeon is 85 to 97 percent.

5. *We conceived our first baby without any problem; the next baby will also be easy.*

Not necessarily. A prior conception is no guarantee that future conceptions will be possible. In both men and women, many factors can intervene to compromise fertility after a successful pregnancy and delivery. For example, a man may develop reproductive tract infections that reduce his sperm quality or ejaculatory function, or the process of labor and delivery may subtly alter the anatomy of a woman's reproductive tract in ways that make a future pregnancy less likely.

6. *If we haven't conceived after one year of trying, we will never get pregnant without IVF.*

Wrong. A couple's inability to conceive is often related to relatively simple or easily corrected problems on the part of either the man or the woman. Couples often wrongly assume that their only option for having children after trying for a year is IVF, when in fact a host of other possible treatments is available, such as clearing up an infection, unclogging the man's ejaculatory ducts, or repairing distended blood vessels in a man's testicles that harm sperm quality. Most of these options are less expensive than IVF. Indeed, in many cases, when these options are pursued first, IVF is more likely to work.

7. *Most couples using IVF end up with a baby.*

Wrong. The unfortunate truth is that the majority of couples undergoing IVF will *not* have a baby. The chance of successful conception and delivery of a baby in a single round of IVF is about 27 percent. The chances of having a baby after two cycles of IVF are about 47 percent—and most couples try for only two cycles because of the expense and emotional strain of the process. The chance of having a baby with IVF after three cycles is about 61 percent, and only after four cycles does it reach about 72 percent.

8. *A man can't do anything to increase his sperm count.*

Wrong. Both the *number* of sperm (sperm count) and the *quality* of that sperm (its shape and function) can be improved. Many men have undiagnosed problems with their testicles or reproductive tract that impair their fertility. Fortunately, such problems are often easily treated, and sperm numbers and quality increase as a result. In addition, moderate exercise, a healthful diet, and avoidance of substances such as cigarettes that are known to erode sperm quality can also improve fertility.

9. *The size of a man's testicles has nothing to do with his fertility, testosterone, and sex drive.*

Wrong. Although the size of a man's penis has little to do with either sexuality or fertility, the size of his testicles does. Testicles are composed of sperm-making and testosterone-producing cells, and generally speaking the larger the testicles, the more sperm and testosterone are produced, which increases sex drive and the chances that a man can get a woman pregnant. Normal testicles are at least the size of walnuts and have the firmness of a ripe plum. Small testicles are the size of cherries or smaller.

10. *Using donor sperm to get pregnant is rare and is certainly used less often than IVF.*

   Wrong. Roughly 40,000 babies in the United States (slightly more than 1 percent of all births) are born each year to couples who have used *in vitro* fertilization techniques of one kind or another. But many more—I estimate about two and a half times as many babies, or about 100,000—are born to women who have conceived using donor sperm, meaning sperm from a sperm bank.

11. *IVF does not increase the chance of birth defects.*

   Wrong. The rate of birth defects in babies born via IVF can be more than two times that of babies conceived naturally.

12. *A low sperm count is not related to a medical condition.*

   Wrong. Testicular cancer, varicoceles, undescended testicles, infection, and chronic illnesses such as diabetes are all associated with low sperm counts.

The unfortunate reality is that infertility is almost always viewed as a "woman's problem" by both the public and many doctors. For academic and business reasons, the entire field of fertility treatment is locked into a mind-set that ignores or marginalizes the male role. A man's fertility is often checked only by a simple semen analysis. If a man seems to have enough sperm and those sperm seem healthy, he is presumed fertile. This kind of cursory "exam" fails to detect a host of problems that could contribute to a fertility problem—most of which can be fixed relatively easily and inexpensively.

The lack of attention to male infertility, the lopsided media and advertising attention paid to female infertility, widespread ignorance about the medical realities of infertility, and the profit motive at work in the infertility industry have combined to create a silent epidemic of infertility. It's probably true that the male ego is involved here too. The possibility of being infertile is deeply threatening to any man's self-esteem and sense of masculinity. This can lead to denial that a problem could exist, defensiveness if the subject is brought up, and a general reluctance to take steps to properly diagnose a potential problem. All these forces have conspired to create an epidemic of male infertility that is going largely unnoticed. Most couples never realize the true dimension of their problem and the often simple steps they could take to remedy the male side of the equation.

The male biological clock affects more than fertility, of course; it affects sexual performance, overall physical health, mental function, and intimate relationships. This book focuses on fertility and sexuality because these are my particular areas of expertise. As the director of male infertility at Columbia University and a board-certified urologist with a large private practice, I have successfully treated many thousands of men with fertility and sexuality problems. I am also a leading researcher on these topics and have participated in dozens of research studies on male infertility over the years. I am privileged to be on the cutting edge of new developments. Over the decades that I have been in this line of work, I have seen firsthand that the male biological clock can be slowed down or even reversed and that problems with sexuality or fertility that arise at any point in a man's life can usually be fixed. This book is about understanding how the clock works, how it can sometimes go awry, and how it can be fixed so a man and his partner can have children or return to an active, satisfying sex life.

A Growing Problem

Men and women are waiting longer to have children and thus have a greater chance of having fertility problems. According to the Centers for Disease Control and Prevention, the number of births to parents older than thirty-five years more than doubled from 1970 to 1999. As the chart below illustrates,

Percentage of Live Births, by Age of Mother

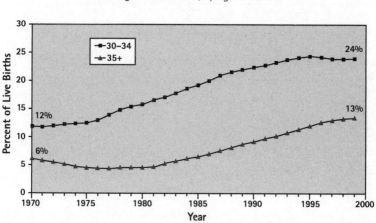

Source: Division of Vital Statistics, National Center for Health Statistics.

over the thirty years, the percentage of live births to women between the ages of thirty and thirty-four doubled, from 12 percent in 1970 to 24 percent in 1999, the last year for which data were available as of this writing. The percentage of live births to women older than thirty-five more than doubled, from 6 percent to 13 percent.

Men are waiting longer to have children too. As the chart below illustrates, the percentage of live births to fathers ages thirty to thirty-four rose from 19 percent to 26 percent from 1970 to 1999. The percentage of births to fathers older than thirty-five rose from 14 percent to 21 percent in the same period.

This trend, coupled with the reality of the male biological clock, have led to the rise in the rates of infertility in the past decade. Each year about 6 million American men and women realize they have a fertility problem. Sadly, most of these cou-

Percentage of Live Births, by Age of Father

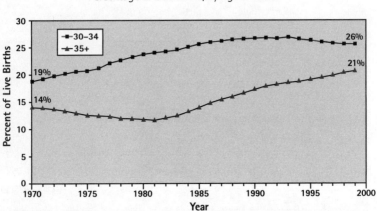

Source: Division of Vital Statistics, National Center for Health Statistics.

ples assume, first, that the problem must be with the woman and, second, that their only option is assisted reproductive technology such as *in vitro* fertilization. Now, don't get me wrong: I'm not against IVF and other assisted reproductive technologies—they are terrific for the right couple at the right time. I help couples through the IVF process all the time, and I've seen many beautiful children come into the world this way. It's just that I've also seen too many couples jump into IVF before they need to, before they've understood all their options, and before the male side of the equation has been thoroughly explored for possible problems.

What *Is* the Male Biological Clock?

Men don't face the absolute end of fertility that women face with menopause. When the female biological clock strikes midnight, a woman's estrogen levels drop precipitously and her ovaries shut down for good. The male biological clock ticks slower and more steadily, and its effects are less obvious. The male equivalent of menopause is "andropause," the steady drop in the levels of androgens (male sex hormones) accompanied by related declines in sperm count, sperm health, sexual desire, and sexual performance. Testosterone is the best-known male hormone, but several others play important roles as well. Changes in male hormones are just as important as changes in female hormones, but currently little attention is given to these changes. The term "andropause" is a somewhat unfortunate one because a man's fertility doesn't, in fact, "pause" the way a woman's does. But "andropause" is better than "hypogonadism in the adult male," which is the technically accurate but fairly clumsy term for what we're talking about. Since "andropause" is commonly accepted and understood by urologists, that's the term I'll use in this book.

How fast and how well a man ages—how fast or slow his "clock" ticks—is governed by his genes, his environment, and how well he takes care of himself. Exactly how the male biological clock works—why some men's clocks run faster than others, for example, or how a man's body "knows" when it's time to move from, say, boyhood to adolescence—is still not entirely clear, but recent research has pinpointed a likely mechanism. The "ticking" of the biological clock of both sexes appears to be linked to cell division. Each time most cells divide, certain caplike sections on the chromosomes inside the cell get a bit shorter. These caps are called telomeres, and they're the subject of intense research around the world, not just because they seem to be involved in the timing of various life stages (such as puberty) but because they may hold the key to aging itself. Certain key cells in the brain are particularly important "timekeepers," and when the telomeres in these cells are whittled down to a certain length, they acquire the ability to turn one's genetic machinery on or off, triggering, for example, the hormonal cascades of adolescence or the shutdown of a woman's ovaries.

Regardless of the actual details, however, neither your

genes nor the clock itself fully determines your destiny. How a man's reproductive tract and sex organs age has everything to do with his overall health: what he eats, how much he exercises, what illnesses and accidents he has sustained in life, whether he smokes or abuses drugs, what chemicals he is exposed to at work or home, and a host of other external factors. The same factors affect female fertility as well, but women usually get years of warning bells about declining fertility, such as irregular periods and hot flashes. (These years are called "perimenopause" and are the lead-in to menopause, which is defined as a year without a menstrual period.)

Problems with sex or fertility are surprisingly common among men and arise from both normal and abnormal functioning of the biological clock. Between 20 and 30 million men have some degree of erectile dysfunction, for example, and despite the huge success of erection-enhancing drugs such as Viagra, Levitra, and Cialis, millions of men continue to suffer. The sex lives of millions of other men are eroded by problems such as premature ejaculation, lack of sexual desire, or the inability to have an orgasm.

This book will help men and their partners understand such problems, determine their source, and lay out a clear path to rewind the biological clock or fix the problems caused by it. Sometimes the steps will be simple and straightforward, such as using an erection-enhancing pill or clearing up an unrecognized infection with antibiotics. Other times more invasive measures must be taken, such as surgery to correct problems in the testicles that affect sperm formation. And sometimes the latest high-tech reproductive technology must be used to overcome obstacles of one kind or another. Regardless of the strategy required, couples should know that most problems with sexuality or fertility can be surmounted.

Viewing male sexual health as the workings of a male biological clock is a new and helpful way of approaching these problems. First, it reminds couples that difficulties with sexuality or fertility are as likely to arise on the male side as the female side of the equation. Acknowledging the reality of the male biological clock creates a level playing field at the outset. No longer is the man merely a bystander, cooling his heels in the waiting room and assuming that *his* anatomy and physiology are perfect while his partner is poked and prodded to uncover a problem assumed to be hers. And even if a problem is found on the woman's side, simply recognizing that it could as easily have been with the man makes it more likely a couple will feel united in their effort to conceive a child.

The facts of the male biological clock also destroy the myth that men of all ages have an equal chance of fathering children. That's simply not true. Recent studies have clearly demonstrated that as men age, the amount and quality of their sperm decline. The declining quality of sperm translates into a lower chance that any particular act of unprotected sex will lead to pregnancy—and that means a longer average time required to get a woman pregnant.

Thinking of male sexual health in terms of a clock also

helps clarify the notion that problems can occur at every stage of life and some problems get progressively worse with time. Infertility or sexual performance problems typically do not happen overnight. They are the end results of circumstances that might have begun at the moment of conception, in childhood or adolescence, or sometimes in adulthood. *Time,* in other words, is a vital part of an accurate view of both the problem and the solution. Problems take time to occur—and they take time to correct. If you are trying to slow or reverse the male biological clock, you have to work *with* the clock; you can't pretend it doesn't exist.

Finally, it's helpful to use a mechanical metaphor for problems of male sexual performance and fertility. Although I realize it's a generalization, I think it's fair to say that most men can relate to machines. Machines can have design flaws that make them likely to break down. Machines also need maintenance if they are to perform well. Both notions apply to male sexuality and fertility problems. And even if a problem is related to choices a man has made about diet, exercise, or drug use, by the time a problem with sexuality or fertility is diagnosed, it's a medical issue—a mechanical breakdown of one sort or another, whether it's as simple as an infection or as subtle as a genetic alteration that is crippling testosterone and sperm production. It is *never* a matter of "manliness" or "machismo."

Every man I've ever known who has learned he has a fertility problem has felt bad—deflated, angry, depressed, or some combination of all of these emotions. That's perfectly normal, given the biological forces driving men to sex and reproduction and the cultural messages supporting those instincts, which are constantly reinforced in the media. But as more men and their partners recognize that they are dealing with a mechanical problem, they'll be able to resist their own (and sometimes others') insinuations that they are somehow to blame for the situation or that they're less of a "man." It's as ludicrous to blame oneself for a low sperm count or hormonal abnormality as it is to blame oneself for having impacted wisdom teeth or being color-blind.

Of course I don't mean to imply that men themselves are machines, just their sexual and reproductive systems. And I'm certainly not saying that sexual performance or fertility problems have no emotional or psychological dimensions. They almost always do—and the emotional knots that can arise from a mechanical breakdown can sometimes be tougher to solve than the breakdown itself! As will be seen throughout this book, I firmly believe in looking at the entire man when dealing with any particular problem. Mind and body cannot be separated. Yes, the specific issue may be a blockage in a man's testicles, but that tiny blockage may be wrecking the emotional and physical intimacy of a previously solid marriage. On the other hand, mental or psychological problems, such as depression or anxiety, can lead to behavior changes (such as exercising less or abusing drugs) that directly erode both sexuality and fertility. Even though in this book we must necessarily concentrate on the mechanical aspects of fertility and sexual performance, and even though I believe the biological clock metaphor is helpful, I don't ever forget that the machinery is inextricably connected to the man as a whole.

Problems with sexual performance or fertility (or both) don't affect just men—they affect their partners as well. Even though the man may have a medical issue that interferes with sex or fertility, his partner is always affected.* Hence this book is aimed at women as much as men. It's women who most often persuade men to seek treatment for infertility or sexual problems. In fact, women persuade men to seek help for practically every physical and mental illness. Women also need to know the facts about male sexual health to be good partners, just as men need to learn the basics of female sexual health. Women may be more objective than their mates in judging the degree to which lifestyle or physical issues can be increasing a man's risk of infertility or sexual performance problems.

I hope that both men and women will find the information and personal stories in this book helpful or perhaps even inspiring. In my daily practice I see much needless suffering caused by a lack of understanding, inaccurate information presented in the media, and misleading claims by fertility clinics. We *are* in an epidemic of unrecognized male infertility and performance problems, but I, for one, am not going to remain silent about it.

---

*Although problems with sexuality affect both heterosexual and homosexual men, a problem with male fertility is by definition, a problem between a man and a woman. Hence throughout this book I tend to use "partner" and "woman" interchangeably, even though I'm certainly aware that sometimes a man's partner is another man.

1
—
The Male
Biological Clock

What Time Is It?

Not all men are created equal biologically. Some men age faster than others. In fact a man's chronological age is actually a poor indicator of the status of his biological clock. Some (admittedly rather rare) eighty-year-old men have sexual and reproductive parameters similar to men fifty years their junior. By the same token, some thirty-year-olds, though they appear fit and healthy, have biological clocks that have been ticking along furiously and have reached a stage more typically seen in men in their seventies. How can a man tell where his biological clock stands? Fortunately, it's relatively simple.

When I say "male biological clock," what I'm talking about is the health status of four of a man's key physical factors:

- Semen
- Sperm
- Testosterone

The "time" shown on a man's particular biological clock is a function of how much semen he ejaculates, how many sperm he produces and how healthy they are, his level of testosterone, and the quality and reliability of his erections. Men scoring high on these measures are biologically young regardless of their age, though, as we'll see, some degradation in the genetic quality of sperm is unavoidable. Many ways exist to improve the four key parameters of sexual health and thus "rewind" (to a certain extent, anyway) the male biological clock in men who score low in any of these areas.

Let's look at these key factors more closely.

Semen

Semen is the milky-colored, somewhat gel-like liquid that spurts out of the penis during orgasm. It is produced not in the testicles, as many men think, but by the small plum-size prostate gland, which sits just below the bladder, and by the seminal vesicles, two pinkie-size glands that feed into the prostate.

Semen is actually a very sophisticated substance. Whole books have been written about it, in fact. Here it's enough to say that it contains nutrients to keep sperm alive after ejacula-

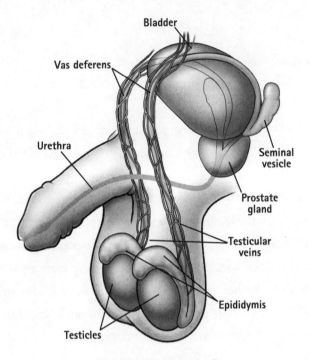

The Male Reproductive Tract

tion, substances to protect the sperm from the chemical environment of the vagina, and special enzymes to make it thin out (liquefy) about fifteen minutes after ejaculation. The average amount (volume) of semen expelled by a healthy man in one ejaculation is about a teaspoon (3 to 5 cubic centimeters). And the semen should spurt or shoot out of the penis, not dribble. Many things in addition to simple aging can reduce the volume of the semen or impair the way it is expelled.

Sperm

A teaspoon of ejaculated semen may not sound like much, but swimming in that teaspoon are usually roughly 250 million sperm, the tadpolelike cells that contain a man's genetic heritage. A healthy man produces sperm at the prodigious rate of about 60,000 every *minute*. But each individual sperm cell takes about three months to grow.

Immature sperm are made in the testicles and then move slowly through a long, tightly coiled tube at the back of each testicle called the epididymis. When they leave the epididymis, they migrate up two thin pipes called the vas deferens. The vas deferens pass through the prostate gland and join the urethra, which is the tube that passes urine from the bladder.

Healthy sperm swim vigorously in a relatively straight line,

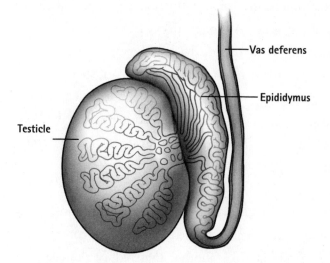

A Testicle, Epididymis, and Lower Part of the Vas Deferens

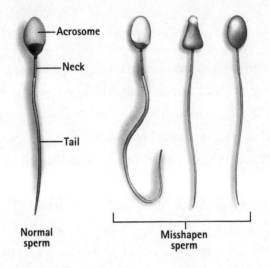

Acrosome

Neck

Tail

Normal
sperm

Misshapen
sperm

Healthy Sperm Compared with Typical Sperm Malformations

their tails are long and whiplike, their heads are well shaped, and the genetic information they carry is intact. Their swimming ability is key. Although an egg in a fallopian tube is only a matter of inches from the back of the vagina, where semen is normally deposited during unprotected sex, sperm are so tiny that the journey is roughly equivalent to a man's running three miles. To reach their target, in other words, they have to swim like crazy. Technically, a sperm's swimming ability is called "motility," and this is a key factor to examine in a good semen analysis.

A sperm's shape is called its "morphology," and it, too, is measured. Abnormally shaped sperm often contain genetic errors of one kind or another that reduce the chances the sperm will fertilize an egg. The more normally shaped sperm there are in his semen, the more likely a man will conceive a healthy child via unprotected sex with a woman.

The number, motility, and shape of sperm all generally decline with age, though many other factors can speed up the biological clock governing this particular facet of a man's overall sexual health.[1] Heat, for example, is bad for sperm. Sperm production plummets in the days following a high fever. Anything that unnaturally warms the testicles, such as taking frequent soaks in a hot tub, will similarly hurt sperm.

The shape of sperm is an indirect measure of the quality of the genetic information they contain, but in recent years it's become possible to directly probe the integrity of the genetic information in individual sperm cells. This is a fairly new field of scientific exploration because it's only recently that the entire human genome has been mapped and techniques for rapidly sampling genetic information have been invented. Research to date clearly shows that a range of genetic problems in sperm get worse with age; these include hemophilia A, neurofibromatosis, Marfan syndrome, and polycystic kidney disease. The graph on the next page shows how the risk of having children with some of the most severe birth defects of all types (so-called sentinel birth defects) rises with the age of the father, particularly when the father is older than thirty-five, which is precisely when more and more couples are having children.

A specific example of this phenomenon is illustrated by a study I worked on that showed that older men are much more likely than younger men to father a child with Down syndrome when their female partner is older than thirty-five. We now know that men contribute to the rising incidence of Down syndrome with age, most likely because the overall incidence of genetic problems in their sperm increases with age. In fact the study found that *half* the cases of Down syndrome in children born to women older than thirty-five are likely to be sperm-related. We now also know that the father's age affects the risk of miscarriage in women older than thirty-five: the older the father, the higher the risk.[2]

The reason the male influence on Down syndrome (as well as other genetic defects and miscarriage) has not been recognized before is that the effect is complicated by the age of the female partner. When a woman is younger than thirty-five, the

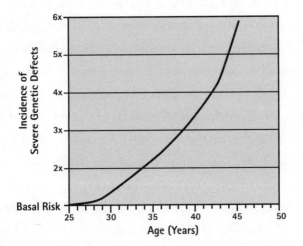

Birth Defects and Paternal Age

age of the man does not seem to affect the overall risk of having a child with Down syndrome, whereas when the woman is older than thirty-five, the age of the man has a pronounced effect. What's going on here? The answer is still being explored, but it seems likely that younger women's bodies are more efficient at detecting and eliminating embryos with genetic problems. In other words, older men are probably conceiving more genetically flawed embryos than younger men, but this fact is masked when the woman is young because the flawed embryos either never implant or are spontaneously aborted.

The ages of *both* partners thus matter when it comes to the risk of having children born with birth defects. As we've seen, there has been a dramatic rise in the age of parents in the past few decades, which could be considered a public health concern because of the increased risk of birth defects that the rise entails. The graph on the next page shows that the number of first-time mothers over thirty-five years of age has increased by 116 percent, and the number of first-time fathers has increased by 50 percent. There has been a less dramatic rise in first-time fathers and first-time mothers between the ages of thirty and thirty-four, while there has been a decline in births to men and women younger than thirty years of age. The hopeful aspect of this situation is that the various techniques for improving the morphology and overall health of sperm that I will discuss later in the book might actually reduce the potential for birth defects by raising the genetic integrity of the chromosomes contained in those sperm.

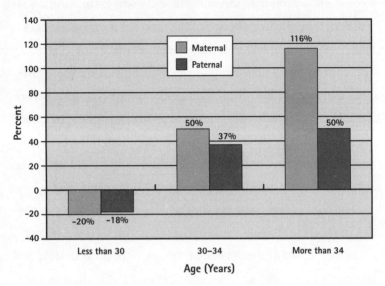

Percentage of Increase in Maternal and Paternal Age
in the United States from 1970 to 1999

Testosterone

A man's biological clock status is also determined by his levels of testosterone, which drives the development of characteristics such as facial hair, muscle development, and interest in sex. Many other hormones play a role in male sexuality, but testosterone is by far the most prominent and the one most often adjusted with supplements of one type or another. (Note that testosterone isn't just a "male" hormone; women have it too. Their average levels are much lower than men's, but testosterone is as central to the female sex drive as it is to the male sex drive. Testosterone also plays a key role in maintaining healthy bones and the cardiovascular system in women. Women with abnormally low testosterone can suffer from a variety of ailments, such as lack of energy and depression, in addition to losing their sexual desire.)

The normal range of testosterone in men is between 300 and 1,100 nanograms (ng) per deciliter (dl) of blood, which is a fairly wide range of "normal" for a bodily component! Levels that fall anywhere in this range confer a normal degree of sexual desire, and they support normal masculine physical and personality traits. Only when men have either very low testosterone levels or very high testosterone levels are physical or mental changes noticeable.

Men with levels below 300 ng/dl (a condition called hypogonadism) tend to have little interest in sex and are usually nonconfrontational, socially inhibited, and physically weak. They are also often very intellectual, creative, expressive, and likable. Men with higher-than-normal testosterone tend to be just the reverse: obsessed with sex, competitive, aggressive, extroverted, physical, and tending toward more action-oriented activities or careers. But within the normal range, testosterone levels play only a background role and other aspects of personality dominate. For example, one study of testosterone levels among actors, ministers, football players, physicians, firefighters, professors, and salesmen found that there was only one statistically significant difference in average testosterone levels—that between ministers (whose average testosterone levels were on the low end) and both actors and football players (whose averages were on the high end).[3] But every group displayed wide individual variations—some football players had lower testosterone levels than some ministers, and some professors had higher testosterone levels than many firefighters.

Whatever a man's basic level, his testosterone level fluctuates widely over the course of a day, peaking in early morning and dropping by 30 to 40 percent by midafternoon.

Testosterone levels usually begin a slow downhill slide of about 1 percent a year starting around age thirty. That loss adds up over the years. Since the average man in the United States can expect to live to age seventy-four, an annual drop of 1 percent means a 44 percent drop in all. More important, men with low-normal testosterone levels (for instance, 400 ng/dl) might hit the threshold of clinically significant testosterone loss by age fifty-five. The signs of below-normal testosterone levels include fatigue, depressed mood, low or absent sex drive, muscle weakness, sleep disorders, and a general feeling of malaise.

Aging, however, isn't the only reason testosterone levels can fall below normal. Here are just a few factors known to reduce testosterone levels at a much faster rate than simple aging:

- Diabetes
- Alcoholism
- Obesity
- Varicoceles

- Use of unprescribed testosterone or other supplements, such as anabolic steroids, that boost testosterone
- Cancer treatments such as chemotherapy and radiation therapy.
- Tumors on the pituitary gland or hypothalamus
- Adult mumps infection
- Chronic illness

This all translates into a serious health problem that is only now beginning to gain widespread recognition. A 2004 article in *The New England Journal of Medicine* estimated that between 2 million and 4 million men in the United States alone have hypogonadism (defined as testosterone levels below 325 ng/dl). The prevalence of hypogonadism clearly increases with age, as the chart below shows. In my experience, men with fertility

Percentage of Men with Low Levels of Bioavailable Testosterone

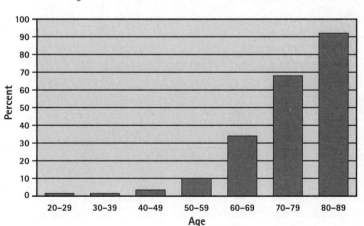

problems are much more likely to have hypogonadism at a young age, indicating a rapid biological clock. In other words, infertile men in their thirties and forties may have testosterone levels of men in their sixties and seventies.

The following chapter explores ways to restore normal levels of testosterone in hypogonadal men. For now, understand that this is another aspect of the male biological clock that can be safely and effectively "rewound" to restore fertility and sex drive, improve muscle strength, reduce fat, and boost overall energy.

Erections

The last measure of a man's sexual health is the quality and reliability of his erections. Erectile dysfunction (formerly called impotence) is the persistent inability to achieve or maintain an

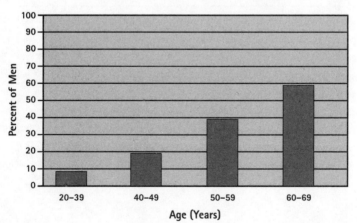

Prevalence of Erectile Dysfunction, by Age

erection adequate for intercourse. It's an enormous problem that has really gotten the attention it deserves only since the introduction in 1998 of the erection-enhancing drug Viagra. The largest study done to date estimates that between 20 million and 30 million men in the United States experience some degree of erectile dysfunction, with the incidence increasing steadily with age.[4]

As with all the other aspects of the male biological clock reviewed earlier in this chapter, erectile dysfunction is caused by an interplay of normal aging and a host of other factors that speed up the biological clock, including the following:

- Smoking
- Diabetes
- Alcohol
- Many prescription medications
- Obesity
- High cholesterol level
- Injury
- Sedentary lifestyle

Basically, what's bad for the heart is bad for the penis. I think if men understood that things like high cholesterol levels put them at greater risk for erectile dysfunction *and* heart disease, they would be more likely to watch their diets, exercise, and seek appropriate help. Fortunately, erectile dysfunction can almost always be successfully treated these days with either medications or a range of other techniques and technologies, detailed in Chapter 3.

Getting Tested

We've looked at the four basic parameters of male sexual health: semen, sperm, testosterone, and erections. Getting a fix on where a man stands—his sexual biological age as opposed to his chronological age—is relatively easy.

A man's testosterone level is checked by drawing a blood sample, usually from the arm. The blood sample should be taken in the morning, since that's when the testosterone level is highest. If the level is below or near 300 ng/dl, another one or two samples may be taken on other days to confirm the first result, since, as noted previously, testosterone levels fluctuate daily and seasonally as well.

Whether or not a man has erectile dysfunction is something he and his partner must judge for themselves based on their personal experience. All men occasionally have problems with their erections. The question is: How often does that happen, and to what degree are the man and his partner bothered by it? These days a man complaining of erectile dysfunction is usually given a trial prescription for an erection-enhancing pill. Only if he can't take the pill because of other risk factors, such as being on a nitrate-containing medication or if the pill fails to work, are more elaborate tests done to try to pinpoint the problem. Such tests can include injection of erection-producing drugs to check the health of the man's penile arteries and veins, and the use of devices that detect the presence and quality of nighttime erections.

The quality of a man's semen and sperm is assessed by a

sample of ejaculate produced by masturbating into a small, sterile plastic container. For some men, this isn't a big deal. They just go to a bathroom in a clinic or doctor's office, do their job, and—presto!—there's a nice, fresh sample that can be analyzed immediately. (Some facilities have private rooms for semen collection that often include erotic magazines or videos to help overcome the unnaturalness of the process.) Other men prefer to masturbate at home and bring their sample to the lab. And some men, for religious reasons, need to collect their semen by having intercourse using a special sterile condom (*not* a standard latex or lambskin condom).

Regardless of how semen is obtained, the sooner it is analyzed, the better. Sperm swim less and less vigorously as the minutes pass after ejaculation. To gauge the vigor of a man's sperm, his semen should not be more than an hour old. In addition, the sample must not be contaminated by other substances or bacteria, which means that men should not have unprotected intercourse to bring themselves to the point of orgasm and should not use artificial lubricants during masturbation.

It's good to plan a semen collection in advance since timing is everything. A man should not "store up" his semen for a long time because sperm in the vas deferens slowly die. If a man doesn't ejaculate for four or five days, his semen will contain more dead sperm than normal. On the other hand, if he has ejaculated one or more times in the past two days, his semen volume will be lower than normal. It's a good idea, therefore, for a man to make sure his last ejaculation was two or three days before the day he collects his semen. (Note: if a man has recently had a high fever or a serious illness or injury, he should talk to his doctor about delaying a semen analysis for about three months to allow his sperm production to recover.)

A sperm count is given as the number of sperm in each milliliter of semen. Healthy men have between 40 million and 300 million sperm per milliliter; the average sperm count is between 60 million and 80 million. Counts below 20 million per milliliter are considered poor and counts between 20 million and 40 million are considered marginal, though possibly fine if other aspects of the sperm, such as their morphology and motility, are good. Men with counts below 20 million may still be fertile, but it may take longer for them to initiate a pregnancy and the chances are greater that a pregnancy will not occur. Men with a high count are not guaranteed to be fertile, however, particularly if an infection or other abnormalities that affect morphology and motility are present.

The graph on the following page illustrates the relationship between sperm counts and both the chances of getting a woman pregnant and the time required to achieve a pregnancy in infertile couples. Each line represents men with a certain sperm count. Men with high counts achieve a pregnancy earlier and are more likely to initiate a pregnancy during any particular act of intercourse.[5]

Interpreting a sperm count correctly requires knowing the total volume of semen in a sample. For example, if a man has 20 million sperm per milliliter of semen, it might be consid-

Relationship Between Sperm Count and Pregnancy Rates

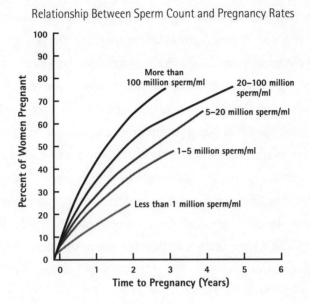

ered low. But if he ejaculates 5 milliliters of semen, his *total* number of sperm would be 100 million—which would be perfectly adequate.

Sperm shape is determined by examining semen under a microscope and counting how many in the small area in view appear normal. Sperm are made in such vast quantities that semen from even the healthiest man contains many dead or misshapen sperm. It's considered normal for as many as 70 percent of the sperm in a sample to be abnormal or dead, though obviously the fewer such sperm there are, the better for fertility.

I want to emphasize that a low sperm count is almost

always the result of some underlying health problem, which can be serious. In other words, a low sperm count is a symptom or clue that something is wrong, not a disease state in and of itself. A low sperm count is like a high fever: the best approach to ameliorating a fever is not to simply take aspirin but to find the underlying problem that is causing the fever and treat that. Not all doctors will tell you that. And many won't pursue the reason for your low sperm count. But *you* should. Some of the most common underlying problems are hormonal irregularities, use of over-the-counter steroids, distended veins in the testicles, diabetes, pituitary tumors, and testicular cancer.

Wrapping Up

The male biological clock starts ticking the moment a sperm containing a male "Y" chromosome successfully fertilizes an egg. If all goes well, roughly nine months later a new baby boy enters the world and begins his journey through life. If he is fortunate, he will live long enough to pass through all the important phases of his biological clock, with all of the pleasures and pains that trip entails.

As we've seen, however, nature doesn't hand out the same clock to everyone. Aside from identical twins, every man is biologically unique. Men (and women) age at different rates due to differences in the details of their biological clocks combined with influences such as diet, stress, exercise, injury, disease, and use of substances (such as cigarettes) that speed aging. Now we've seen how to determine what "time" a man's biological clock is tolling: a blood test for testosterone, a semen analysis, and a determination by a man and his partner of the quality of his erections.

But even though a man's own particular biological clock sets broad limits on his sexuality and fertility, we now know how to offset, reverse, or overcome almost all problems in those two areas. Understanding the ways in which genes, aging, and lifestyle factors can erode sexual health is the first step to doing something about it. We'll now take a closer look at specific ways to rewind the clock, starting with the issue of how to treat low hormone levels in men.

2

The Truth About Testosterone

After his wife was checked out for fertility problems and nothing untoward was found, Jason, her husband, went for a semen analysis.

"Jane was checked out first because, of course, it's always the woman's problem, right?" he said. "But it turned out it was me—I had no sperm and a low testosterone level."

When Jason, who was forty, came to see me, I confirmed his testicular failure, and also found a testicular tumor that required removal of that testicle. That left Jason with even less ability to make testosterone.

Eventually, he and his wife had two children using *in vitro* fertilization and a technique for finding sperm and injecting them directly into a woman's eggs (discussed fully in Chapter 5).

But Jason's story isn't about his wife's successful delivery of healthy twins. It's about the effects of the testosterone therapy that he has now used for five years. In order to treat Jason's extremely low testosterone levels (they were in the range of a sixty-year-old man), he began a course of testosterone injections every two weeks in order to boost his testosterone level to the normal range.

"I was about a hundred pounds overweight," Jason says. "I had been through every diet in the book, and the weight always came back. But the testosterone gave me a boost of energy that I never had before, and for some reason, to this day, it allows me to control my appetite."

At my suggestion, Jason began eating a sensible, healthy diet, and once he began to feel the testosterone kick in, he began to exercise for the first time in his life.

"When people would talk about their endorphins kicking in and getting that high from exercise, I didn't know what they were talking about," Jason says. "But now I do. With the testosterone, your body feels high, like you've got huge energy. You're not sluggish, you sleep better, you bounce out of bed, take a shower, and you want to get to work. It's that kind of feeling. Mind you, sometimes it's still drudgery to go to the gym, but once I'm there, I really enjoy it, whereas before I could never even dream of exercising like this."

Jason lost more than ninety pounds. He could buy clothes off the rack for the first time instead of having them custom made. He became much more confident in himself and says he feels years younger.

"Did it change my personality?" he asks. "Maybe. But I lost ninety pounds at the same time, so is it the weight loss or the testosterone? I don't know."

Jason is president of a thriving small business. He recalls a time after he'd lost his weight and bought new clothes. He had a meeting with a company that was threatening to sever its ties with his business.

"They were saying they didn't want to work with us, but I lost my weight and went into that meeting with my new look, Gucci suit, hip, no tie, open shirt, but in a conservative sort of way, and it was completely different," he says. "I turned the whole thing around. And they're one of our biggest accounts now. Because the perception of me changed. I was no longer this person who looked overweight and tired. All of a sudden I was a person with much more confidence, and I'm more gutsy, more full of myself."

Like most men who use testosterone replacement therapy, Jason notices a distinctly heightened sex drive, particularly in the first few days after an injection. Although he says he's never had a problem with his erections, now, at forty-four, he has noticed that his erections are more robust and he's more easily aroused with testosterone.

Jason uses his testosterone responsibly and maintains his levels in the mid-normal range. He gets blood tests every six months to monitor his liver function and prostate health.

Thus far, he is much healthier now than before he began. His cholesterol levels and blood pressure improved and are excellent. And he has experienced an unexpected benefit: relief from panic attacks.

"My panic attacks were so severe that I couldn't get on a plane without getting drunk and having my pills," he says. "It got to the point that I couldn't even be in open places. But I haven't had an attack now in four years. I'm in control now—and that's the problem with panic, you feel like you're out of control. The shot makes me feel like I'm in control."

Of course, testosterone therapy, particularly with injections, isn't without drawbacks. Jason, who tried but just can't give himself an injection, must make regular visits to get his shots, which can be a problem when he travels.

"It's a hassle," he says. "You know, getting to the nurse, 'Which cheek will it be this week?' It's a pain in the neck."

He's also not thrilled that he expects to have to continue this routine the rest of his life. Although new methods for delivering testosterone have been developed since Jason began his therapy, they don't give him the level he finds works best. Still, he says the hassle and discomfort are worth it.

"Heart disease runs in my family," he says. "My dad died at forty-seven. I was overweight and never would have lost that weight without the testosterone. Never. Now my cholesterol is incredible. I exercise hard at least three times a week. And isn't it healthier and better to be like this than to have been going on the track I was before, which I'm sure would have led to a serious problem?"

A Growing Problem *and* a Dangerous Fad

Changes in men's hormones are just as important as changes in women's hormones. Between 2 million and 4 million men in the United States alone suffer from below-normal testosterone levels, a condition known as hypogonadism.[1] It's a problem that gets progressively more common as men age, though it can strike men at any age for a variety of reasons. Unfortunately, very few men with below-normal testosterone are getting the help they need. It's estimated that only 5 percent of the millions of men with hypogonadism are currently being treated, despite a booming business in testosterone replacement therapies of many kinds. (Sales of prescription testosterone products have soared by more than 500 percent since 1993.)[2] This surge in the use of testosterone products may not be an entirely good thing. Testosterone replacement therapy is appropriate and safe *only* for men like Jason who have a below-normal level and who don't have any medical conditions that could be made worse by testosterone, such as an enlarged prostate or evidence of prostate cancer. As we'll see, use of testosterone by men with a normal level is very risky.

The symptoms of hypogonadism are often overlooked, in part because they are mistaken for ordinary signs of aging. Men with below-normal testosterone experience the following:

- Low interest in sex
- Fatigue
- Sleep disturbance
- Muscle weakness
- Small or soft testicles
- Erectile dysfunction
- Weight gain, particularly around the waist
- Reduced bone density (osteoporosis)
- Depression
- Anemia

The enormous industry that has sprung up to capitalize on this problem has contributed to a dangerous rise in the unregulated sale and use of testosterone supplements. Far too many men are obtaining quick-and-dirty prescriptions for testosterone and abusing the hormone because it makes them feel temporarily younger and stronger. Myths and misunderstandings about testosterone abound. Here are the ones I hear most frequently.

1. *Testosterone replacement improves fertility.*

   False. As we will see in this chapter, inappropriate use of testosterone—such as how it may be used by athletes for performance enhancement—can effectively sterilize a man and cause his testicles to shrink and become soft. Stimulating the body's *own* production of testosterone, on the other hand, *can* improve fertility.

2. *Being overweight has nothing to do with testosterone levels.*

Wrong. Extra fat on the body acts like a sponge, taking testosterone out of the blood and reducing libido, energy, and other male-related characteristics. This is particularly true if the fat is carried around the belly or abdomen. Fat carried on the thighs or buttocks has less of a testosterone-draining effect.

3. *Men can raise their testosterone level by exercising vigorously.*

Yes, but the relationship between testosterone and exercise is complicated. Exercise can raise the testosterone level somewhat, but if exercise is extreme, the testosterone level can actually drop. It's also true that low testosterone makes it harder to exercise, which can lead to a vicious cycle of inactivity and reduced hormone levels.

4. *Male midlife crises have nothing to do with testosterone.*

I believe that many times when men say they are bored with their careers, their wives, or their general lot in life, they are actually suffering from low testosterone. I call this phenomenon "menoporsche" because I've seen guys who think buying a hot new car like a Porsche will give them a shot of sex appeal or attractiveness, when, in fact, they would be much better off getting their testosterone level checked.

5. *Testosterone supplements are safe because they have to be approved by the FDA.*

Wrong. In fact, as of this writing, the government does *not* regulate the sale or use of products containing compounds that are converted into testosterone. Testosterone or testosterone precursors should be used only under a doctor's supervision and testosterone should be raised only to the normal level.

6. *Low testosterone causes depression.*

True, but that's just half the story. Most men don't know that depression, or depressed mood, can lower their testosterone level. Since many men don't recognize the signs that they are depressed or are reluctant to seek help in treating their depression, this is a significant problem for millions of men. Sometimes restoring a man's testosterone level can also alleviate his symptoms of depression—and sometimes alleviating the depression with psychotherapy and/or antidepressant medications can raise testosterone levels.

7. *Erection-enhancing medications such as Viagra work whether a man has normal testosterone levels or not.*

In fact, studies show that erection-enhancing medications work best in men with testosterone levels in the normal range. Testosterone also provides the necessary urge to have sex that erection-enhancing drugs cannot provide.

8. *Testosterone therapy is really just a form of cosmetic pharmacology— it's just something middle-aged men try to make themselves feel young.*

Wrong. Testosterone replacement for men of any age who have a below-normal level is a valid medical treatment for a condition with the clear potential to degrade overall health and well-being. Failure to treat hypogonadism puts men at higher risk for frailty, osteoporosis, heart disease, and, perhaps, Alzheimer disease.

9. *Low testosterone is a problem only for old men.*

False. Certainly, the older you are, the more likely you are to have low testosterone, but this condition can affect any man, even a teenager. Conditions such as varicoceles, undescended testicles, and certain genetic problems can cause below-normal testosterone levels, which need to be diagnosed and corrected as quickly as possible.

10. *The only way to boost testosterone levels is with shots or gels.*

False. A potentially better approach is to coax the body to increase testosterone levels naturally rather than by dumping testosterone directly into the bloodstream by shots, gels, or patches. In most men, this can be done by pills that stimulate the brain to increase the production of testosterone from the testicles.

Being Smart About Testosterone

Testosterone clearly plays a major role in men's health and fertility, but achieving a healthy level must be done the right way. As with anything, knowledge is power, and to reap the benefits of testosterone therapy you must learn a little about what testosterone is, how it works, and what can cause its level to sink below normal.

Low testosterone (hypogonadism) can be caused by many factors, all of which play out against the normal steady decline in testosterone level with age. Tumors on the pituitary gland (which controls testosterone production in the testicles), problems with the testicles themselves, injury, infections, and being overweight can all cause testosterone to drop below normal levels. Excess body fat does this because testosterone is normally broken down in the body's fat cells; hence, if you have a lot of fat, your body breaks down testosterone extra-quickly, leading to a deficiency. And, as mentioned on page 44, abdominal or "belly" fat has a greater capacity to break down testosterone than other types of fat.

Another risk factor for hypogonadism that has only recently come to light is diabetes. A strong relationship has been discovered between impaired glucose tolerance, which is a cardinal feature of diabetes, and low testosterone levels. It appears that the high blood sugar levels and/or low insulin levels characteristic of diabetes harms the cells in the testicles that are responsible for making testosterone. A very recent study of 221 middle-aged men confirmed this finding: the men most likely to be diabetic also had the lowest testosterone levels.[3]

The reverse may also occur: a low testosterone level may decrease insulin sensitivity to lower muscle mass, thereby making diabetes worse. Because diabetes, particularly adult-onset diabetes, has been steadily rising as a health problem in most developed countries, the prevalence of hypogonadism associated with this disorder will likely rise as well in coming years. We've already seen a rise in a condition known as metabolic syndrome, which is a prediabetic state among men that includes low testosterone level, abnormal lipid profile, insulin insensitivity, and weight gain around the middle. In fact, one of the clearest signs of both low testosterone and a tendency toward diabetes is abdominal fat. If your waist is larger than 40 inches and you tend to carry excess weight in your middle, as opposed to your thighs or buttocks, you may be at risk for both conditions.

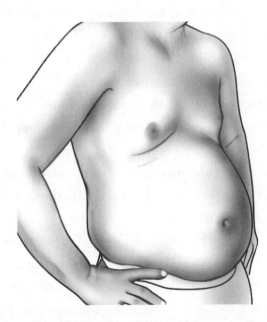

Abdominal fat is linked to low testosterone levels.

Why Testosterone Replacement Isn't for Everyone

Many body tissues are sensitive to testosterone, including the muscles, bones, brain, skin, testicles, blood, and prostate gland. This means that any alteration in testosterone level will have very wide-ranging effects. For men with truly inadequate testosterone, increasing testosterone may be a boon—or at least the risks are outweighed by the potential benefits of therapy. For men with normal testosterone levels, though, increasing testosterone is hazardous.

The most familiar risk from boosting testosterone is raising the risk of prostate cancer or prostate enlargement. In truth, the latest research can't pin down this risk very well because the necessary long-term controlled clinical trials have not been done. In a very real sense, medicine is at the same stage with testosterone replacement therapy (TRT) in men as it was with hormone replacement therapy (HRT) for women twenty years ago. That should be a red flag for everyone involved in the current debates over TRT. When hormone replacement therapy was first used with women, it was considered to be very safe and to have many positive attributes, such as being good for the heart and bones. Early, short-term, and preliminary studies seemed to bear this out. But when long-term studies were eventually done, it became clear that HRT not only increases the risk of certain cancers, it is *not* beneficial for the heart. Because of all this, other treatments are now being used for alleviating menopausal symptoms, increasing bone density, and ensuring female cardiovascular health.

The suggestion that testosterone replacement therapy may increase the risk of prostate problems comes from several related lines of evidence. First of all, we know that the prostate is very sensitive to testosterone levels—testosterone causes prostate growth, while its elimination shrinks the prostate. In fact, various methods of reducing testosterone are used to treat both prostate cancer and benign prostate enlargement. Studies also clearly demonstrate that the prostate grows following testosterone supplementation. Prostate enlargement, by itself, is not necessarily a problem; it's only when that growth causes pain or other problems, such as difficulty urinating or an inability to empty the bladder fully that it needs to be treated. The studies to date have failed to find a correlation between testosterone replacement therapy and annoying urinary symptoms that sometimes—but not always—accompany enlargement.[4]

A less well-known effect of boosting testosterone is an increase in the numbers of oxygen-carrying red blood cells. Again, for men suffering from anemia or lack of energy, this effect may be welcome and can increase their energy and endurance. But adding blood cells also makes the blood thicker and more prone to clogging in tiny vessels; hence it can theoretically increase the risk of a variety of cardiovascular problems, such as heart attack and stroke.

One original concern about the safety of testosterone therapy has dissipated in recent years. Early studies suggested that testosterone replacement therapy hurt the balance of high-density lipoprotein (the so-called good cholesterol) to low-density lipoprotein (the "bad" cholesterol). But more recent studies suggest that as long as the testosterone level is held within normal limits, the blood lipid profile is unaffected or may even improve.

Testosterone replacement therapy can sometimes cause other, less potentially serious effects, such as increased acne, increased snoring and sleep apnea (sudden waking from a transitory interruption of breathing), softening of the testicles, and breast tenderness or enlargement. It may also speed up male-pattern baldness, though this effect has not been rigorously documented.

Whether fertility is affected by testosterone replacement therapy depends on many factors. As a general rule, male infertility can be caused by low testosterone, but boosting testosterone artificially usually *reduces* fertility even more. In fact, a relatively high level of testosterone acts as a fairly effective form of birth control.

This fact is not widely known, and *thousands of men are using testosterone supplements that hurt their fertility.*

Steve was one of those guys. When Steve came to see me, he was wearing a tight-fitting polo shirt that revealed a heavily muscled torso. He was tan and gave the outward appearance of excellent health. But he had practically no sperm in his semen, and his testicles were small and soft. My suspicion that he was using a supplement that boosted his testosterone was confirmed when his blood test results came back: his testosterone level was three times higher than normal.

Here's how all that extra testosterone had essentially crippled his reproductive system.

A man's body (actually, certain key parts of his brain) constantly monitors the level of testosterone in his blood. When the level falls the brain sends signals to the testicles to boost production, and when the level rises, the brain tells the testicles to shut down. Adding extra testosterone, in other words, tricks the brain and causes it to send signals that shut down not only testosterone production but sperm production as well. The result is smaller, softer testicles and infertility.

When I explained this to Steve, he was shocked. He had no idea. He agreed to stop taking the supplements he was using, and I prescribed a medication to help kick-start his body's natural testosterone production machinery. His sperm count began to come back in three months, and by six months it was normal. Several months after that, Steve's wife became pregnant and later delivered a healthy baby girl.

Steve's case illustrates the potential hazards of testosterone on fertility. We'll talk more about over-the-counter products later, but here I want to stress that if you are trying to have a baby, do not use any nutritional or natural supplements that claim they will boost muscle mass, increase your metabolism, or promote growth. All such products can hurt your fertility, ejaculatory function, or erectile function.

In certain cases, however, judicious manipulation of testosterone can improve sperm counts, motility, and morphology. This is best done, in my opinion, by using medications that indirectly boost the body's production of testosterone rather than using testosterone replacement itself. (See the section on alternatives to testosterone later in this chapter.)

The bottom line is that testosterone replacement therapy is a real, potentially valuable treatment for men with below-normal levels, but it poses equally real risks for men with normal levels. Any man considering testosterone replacement therapy of any kind *must* have his prostate checked beforehand, with both a digital rectal exam and a blood test for his level of prostate-specific antigen (PSA), which is a marker of prostate health. Any man already using testosterone replacement therapy should have these tests done every six months.

Types of Testosterone Replacement Therapy

Testosterone molecules are rapidly destroyed in the acidic conditions of the stomach and are therefore poorly absorbed. When taken orally, testosterone also impacts the liver, sometimes dangerously. For these reasons, testosterone pills, though available, are not recommended by most doctors in this country. The safest ways to deliver testosterone avoid the stomach, entering instead through the skin via gels or patches or directly into the blood via injections. These approaches differ in how well they create an even, natural level of testosterone. Injections, which are done every two to three weeks, produce a very spiky pattern of testosterone levels.

Injection results in an above-normal level immediately

Testosterone Levels Typically Produced by Injection

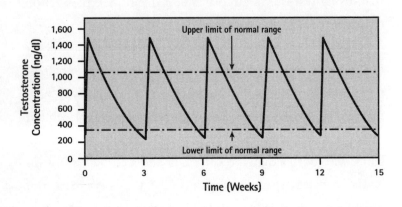

after the injection and a below-normal level in the days before the next injection. Injections come in a variety of doses and are usually given every two to three weeks. In addition to the erratic testosterone level they produce, injections are somewhat painful and involve frequent trips to a doctor's office if a man is not willing or able to inject himself. Side effects from testosterone injections are relatively uncommon but can include acne or oily skin, sleep apnea (temporary cessation of breathing during sleep, which prompts waking), breast swelling, and softening or shrinking of the testicles.

Patch and gel forms of testosterone, by contrast, produce much more steady and even levels of testosterone, as you can see in the graph on the next page.

The gel form of testosterone is the newest and, as of this writing, the most popular way to deliver testosterone. It is also

Testosterone Levels Produced by Patch or Gel

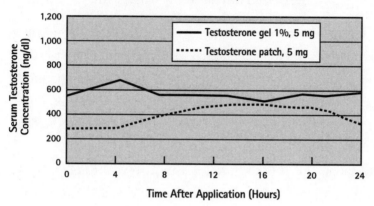

the best way to maintain an even hormone level and reduce undesirable side effects such as those just mentioned above for injections. Patches and gels may cause skin irritation, and gels have the potential side effect of causing inadvertent transfer of testosterone to others who rub against the gel. Sold under the brand name AndroGel, this preparation is a clear, quick-drying gel containing 1 percent testosterone. Applied daily on the skin of the upper arm, shoulders, or abdomen, it begins releasing testosterone through the skin in about thirty minutes.

Two types of testosterone patches are available, one of which is applied to the scrotum, the other to the back, stomach, thighs, or upper arms. The patches share the advantage of the gel in delivering a steady, even dose of testosterone to the body, though they are significantly more likely to cause skin irritation or a rash.

An Alternative to Testosterone

Clomiphene citrate, marketed in pill form as Clomid or Serophene, has long been used for female infertility to spur the ovaries to produce mature eggs. It works by stimulating a part of the brain (the pituitary gland) that controls production of two hormones that are essential to reproductive health: follicle-stimulating hormone (FSH) and luteinizing hormone (LH). Both hormones are also vital to men. FSH stimulates sperm production in the testicles, and LH stimulates testosterone production. So it made sense to a number of urologists who treat male infertility, including me, to try clomiphene citrate in men. A number of studies have now conclusively demonstrated that this strategy works—and it does so by working *with* the body rather than dumping extra testosterone on it from outside. The result? A much-reduced risk of impaired fertility. Indeed, judicious use of clomiphene citrate can stimulate sperm production and sperm quality in men with reduced testicular function.

For example, Murray came to me because he and his wife were having difficulty getting pregnant and a semen analysis showed he had a low sperm count. When I examined him, I found a varicocele (pronounced "VAYR-uh-ko-seal"), which is a set of distended veins in the testicles. Varicoceles are a common cause of impaired fertility because the extra blood in the veins around a testicle warms the testicle, which hurts the cells that produce sperm. (See Chapter 4 for more information about diagnosing and treating varicoceles.)

After surgically repairing the varicocele, I prescribed Clomid to boost Murray's testosterone levels, which, in turn, usually helps sperm production. About six months after the surgery, Murray's sperm counts had improved and his wife got pregnant. Unfortunately, she had a miscarriage, but she got pregnant again soon after and carried the child to term. Their little boy was born ten weeks ago as of this writing.

The Clomid raised Murray's testosterone level, and he liked how he felt on it. An avid runner, he noticed significant changes in his strength and energy.

"I felt more energized and stronger," he says. "I noticed that I could do more pull-ups, and my running times kept going down. I was running with more motivation and strength."

Murray noticed an increase in his mood and his sex drive. The only side effects he noticed were some insomnia in the initial weeks of the treatment and a tendency to sweat more easily, particularly on his palms. He liked the feeling the Clomid gave him so much, he decided to stay on it after his wife got pregnant.

Murray's story is backed up by solid research. Here's an example of the kind of data published on the use of clomiphene citrate:

A group of 178 men with below-normal levels of testosterone were studied.[5] Their average testosterone level at the start of the study was about 250 ng/dl. The men were randomly assigned to receive either clomiphene or a placebo (dummy pill). After four months, the testosterone levels in the clomiphene group had doubled, while the levels in the placebo group had not risen significantly. Seventy-five percent of the men on clomiphene also reported increased libido and sexual functioning.

It's important to point out that some of the warnings and caveats about testosterone mentioned above also apply to clomiphene. This treatment should be used *only* by men with below-normal testosterone and only by men who are not at risk for prostate cancer, cardiovascular problems, stroke, or breast cancer. Men using clomiphene therapy still need to be regularly monitored for prostate problems with both a PSA test and digital rectal exam. These are sensible precautions, since we're still in the early stages of research on this medication in men.

I believe that using clomiphene is an excellent way to raise the body's testosterone level, particularly by men who are using it to treat infertility. Other drugs similar to clomiphene are being developed that may provide similar benefits with, perhaps, lower risks (though clomiphene is, relatively speaking, a very safe drug). These drugs are called selective estrogen receptor modulators, or SERMs, and, like clomiphene, they work by stimulating a man's body to make more testosterone. Future research into these drugs and others like them may provide a new generation of medications that will safely and effectively increase testosterone levels without the need for direct testosterone replacement therapy.

Other Hormones

As just mentioned, testosterone isn't the only important hormone involved in male sexual health. The regulation of both testosterone levels and sperm production starts with a master control gland in the brain called the hypothalamus. The hypothalamus secretes gonadotropin-releasing hormone (GnRH), which travels to the nearby pituitary gland and stimulates that gland to make two other key hormones: luteinizing hormone, which controls testosterone production, and follicle-stimulating hormone, which stimulates sperm production.

Sometimes the hypothalamus gland is damaged by a tumor, radiation, or unknown reasons and doesn't produce enough GnRH —a condition with the tongue-twisting name "hypothalamic-hypogonadotropic hypogonadism." With the master control switched off, the pituitary never gets the signal to produce its hormones and the testicles remain in a juvenile state, producing neither testosterone nor sperm. Treatment with a combination of twice-weekly injections of a compound called "human chorionic gonadotropin," coupled with another medication called Pergonal to boost sperm production, frequently restores normal functioning and fertility. GnRH itself can also be delivered via a portable infusion pump that delivers the hormone directly to the bloodstream every two hours.

The pituitary gland is also subject to failure, most commonly as a result of a noncancerous benign hormone-secreting tumor such as prolactinomas. Prolactin is normally found in very low levels in men but high levels in women, where it stimulates milk production in the breasts. Pituitary tumors or genetic defects in the pituitary can send the prolactin level soaring, producing a range of symptoms such as low sperm count, loss of sexual desire, trouble reaching orgasm, and growth of breast tissue around the nipples. High prolactin levels in a man also disrupt the actions of other reproductive hormones, which, in turn, further hurts fertility. Treatment with the medication bromocriptine or Dostinex often succeeds in restoring a normal hormone level and fertility. It can also shrink pituitary tumors. Side effects of the drug include fatigue in the early stages of treatment, headache, nausea, and dizziness.

Here are the normal levels for all the important hormones related to male sexuality:

Testosterone	300–1,100 ng/dl
FSH	0.8–9 mIU/ml
LH	0.5–10 mIU/ml
Prolactin	0.1–15.2 ng/dl

The specific pattern of abnormalities (if any) in these hormones can help determine if a problem is in the testicles, the pituitary gland, or other parts of the brain or body.

Over-the-Counter Products

In the quest for bigger muscles, improved athletic performance, or enhanced sexuality, hundreds of thousands of men
have turned to over-the-counter compounds that purport to
boost testosterone. Some of these products are actually fake
versions of FDA-approved products such as testosterone
patches or gels. Others contain compounds that are converted to testosterone in the body. The most common of
these testosterone precursors are dehydroepiandrosterone
(DHEA) and androstenedione. The latter gained notoriety
in the late 1990s, when baseball slugger Mark McGwire dis-
closed that he routinely used "andros" (though he didn't say
how *much* he used).

Scientific studies of both precursors using recommended
doses of 100 to 300 mg a day have failed to prove any of the
sometimes outlandish claims made by their manufacturers.[6]
Nonetheless, many anecdotal reports suggest that some men
do indeed see results from these compounds, such as added
strength and bigger muscles. The explanation for the discrep-
ancy is undoubtedly that many men are using doses far higher
than those suggested by the manufacturers and higher than
those used in the scientific studies.

The bottom line: precursor compounds do end up as
testosterone, and thus all of the risks noted above apply to
them. It doesn't matter that the testosterone is produced by
the body in this case—the extra testosterone will impair fer-

tility, bring a man's natural testosterone production to a screeching halt, and increase his risk for prostate cancer, heart attack, and stroke.

The safest approach is simply to avoid *all* nutritional supplements if you are trying to have a baby because many contain hormones or hormone precursors that can hurt fertility and ingredients are often labeled in deceptive ways. The array of products now available is so huge and the number of brand names so large that a comprehensive list isn't feasible. In general, however, any supplement containing the following ingredients or including the following words should be suspect:

- Testosterone
- Dehydroepiandrosterone (DHEA)
- Androstenedione
- Androstenediol
- Prohormone
- Prehormone
- Hormone
- Anabolic

Men should also avoid any products that claim to boost energy because they often contain stimulating compounds such as ephedra, caffeine, and analogs of amphetamine. Such stimulants can impair ejaculatory function and reduce the amount of semen ejaculated at orgasm. Compounds containing human growth hormone (HGH) or claiming to boost growth hormone should be avoided as well, by the way. Research on the potential effects of such products on fertility has not been done, but we do know that such hormones stimulate *all* growth in the body—including the growth of both cancerous and noncancerous tumors.

In summary, abnormally low testosterone—one of the cardinal signals of an advanced biological clock—can safely be increased for the millions of men suffering from hypogonadism. Men on testosterone replacement therapy can realistically look forward to renewed interest in sex, improved erectile function, and (if they also exercise) larger and stronger muscles and reduced fat. The erosion of sexual performance wrought by the clock can thus be remedied quite effectively. Always bear in mind that the use of testosterone or any of the many products containing testosterone precursors by men with normal levels can be dangerous and will likely hurt their fertility. Before beginning testosterone replacement therapy, men should attend to all the factors reviewed in Chapter 6 to improve their overall health and fitness.

3

Viagra Generation

Norm had a great life: wife, two kids, dog, nice home in a small town, and satisfying work. The only thing he didn't have, it seemed, was sex.

Like many couples, Norm's sex life with his wife, Margaret, had evolved from the passion-filled, playful, and lusty days of courtship, to the regular and satisfying sex of early marriage, through long sexless stretches in the aftermath of the births of their children. Now, as he was approaching fifty, sex was so infrequent he usually couldn't remember the last time he and his wife had made love.

Age and the sheer familiarity of sex with his wife played a role in Norm's situation, but he also suspected another cause: his unpredictability as a lover.

Even in the early days of his marriage, Norm would occasionally lose his erection, usually during foreplay as he was helping his wife get aroused and lubricated. Often, by the time she was ready, he was limp.

"It's just awful to have my wife lying there, ready and willing, and not be able to get an erection," he says. "She said she understood, but I'm not sure she did and she was probably as frustrated by it as I was."

The problem would come and go. Sometimes (often after he had a drink or two) he wouldn't worry about his erection and sex would be, if not wild, at least mutually satisfying. But equally often, it seemed, his fear of losing his erection made it impossible for him to achieve one. Over the years, he initiated sex less and less often—and with the addition of children the excuses were easy to find.

"When you have kids, you're often both so exhausted that it's really just easier not to have sex," Norm says. "The thing is, I really *wanted* to have sex. Hell, when I masturbated I had no problems with erections. But when it came to sex with Maggie—I just wasn't confident. I'm sure she felt that, and I'm also sure it's not exactly attractive."

When Viagra became available, Norm didn't consider trying it. He figured he wouldn't be a candidate since he could, after all, get erections on his own. He didn't see himself as having erectile dysfunction even though his history suggested a less-than-robust erectile capacity. But one day a fight with Maggie over who did more housework escalated and suddenly veered into her dissatisfaction with their sex life.

"She said at one point, 'I'm just not attracted to you sometimes, and the fact that you can't make love to me doesn't help.' That's when I decided to give the pill a try. I think we'd both been pretending that sex wasn't really very important to us. We'd been married for sixteen years, we snuggled together in bed, and we basically had a good relationship. But underneath, we were obviously both angry and frustrated."

The first time he popped the little blue pill, Norm was skeptical.

"I really didn't think it was going to work," he says. "And also it had been so long since Maggie and I made love that the whole thing felt a little strange."

But it did work.

"I got an erection very easily," Norm says. "I started to go too fast for Maggie . . . I was so used to feeling like I had to penetrate her or I'd lose my erection. So I slowed down, and relaxed, and I was amazed that the erection just stayed there. It was great. Like the old days—maybe better."

In the year since that first trial with Viagra, Norm says he and Maggie have made love roughly once a week, using the pill every time.

"That may not sound like much to some guys," he says, "but it's just right for me, and I think for Maggie too. I've been struggling for years with a self-image that I'm not a very good lover. I may still not be Casanova, but I'm a helluva lot more confident now than in the past."

The Pill Redux

Stories like Norm's have become quite common. Introduced in 1998, Viagra has become one of the blockbuster drugs of the twenty-first century. About 16 million men have taken Viagra since it was introduced. In 2003 alone, the drug company Pfizer sold $1.7 billion worth of Viagra. And it's not just older men with erection problems who are using the pills. An unknown number of younger men are using Viagra or one of the two new entries to the market, Levitra and Cialis, to enhance their normal erections, to reduce performance anxiety, or simply to experiment.

This widespread public acceptance isn't surprising since Pfizer has poured hundreds of millions of dollars into advertising and promotion—almost $90 million in the year 2000 alone. Similar pushes can be expected from the manufacturers of Levitra and Cialis, and sales of these pills are likely to skyrocket in coming years.

Until recently, some research suggested that the already huge market for these pills might double because they treat female sexual dysfunction as well. But after spending eight years and millions of dollars, Pfizer pulled the plug on its research into the utility of Viagra in women. It turns out that although a woman's clitoris responds in a similar way to a man's penis and Viagra does enhance clitoral engorgement, this did not translate into clinically significant improvement in sexual function, such as the ability to achieve an orgasm or an increased desire for sex. A few very preliminary studies, however, find that if Viagra is combined with a low dose of testosterone replacement therapy, the results for women are very satisfactory. That is undoubtedly because the testosterone boosts a woman's libido while the Viagra increases such things as vaginal lubrication, clitoral response, and other physical aspects of sexual arousal.

As someone who has seen firsthand the kind of grief that can accompany erectile dysfunction, you might think I'd be pleased that erection-enhancing drugs are so widely used. In fact, I think these pills are being overprescribed, overused, and used by men who don't have a clue about the real cause of their erectile dysfunction.

I'm worried that men are being prescribed Viagra and its cousins without a proper search for medical conditions such as diabetes and heart disease that may be causing the erectile problems. Failing erections can be like a dying canary in a coal mine—an early sign of a significant medical problem. Several studies have shown a very high correlation, for example, between erectile dysfunction and the risk of heart attack or stroke. Fixing a failing erection without checking for potentially important underlying problems is like taking a painkiller for a toothache. The solution is to take care of the tooth, not just mask the pain with drugs.

I'll look at these drugs in detail in a moment, but first it's important for both men and women to understand how erections work and why they sometimes fail.

The Clock and Erections

The penis has a mind of its own. It can be coaxed, it can be wooed, and it can be enticed, but it cannot be ordered. As Leonardo da Vinci observed of the male organ, "Many times the man wishes it to practice and it does not wish it; many times it wishes it and the man forbids it." All men, of course, experience times when an erection fails, whether because of stress, tiredness, one drink too many, or just the unpredictable nature of sexual arousal itself. But aging—the male biological clock—definitely takes a toll on erections. That's because, fundamentally, an erection is a matter of plumbing, hydraulics, chemistry, and nerve impulses, all of which depend on physical structures that wear out, to one degree or another, as a man ages. Fortunately, of the many ways the male biological clock can degrade sexual health, its impact on erections is today the most readily corrected.

Erectile dysfunction usually begins as a purely physical problem with blood vessels, nerves, or other parts of the male reproductive machinery. But very rapidly a complicated psychological dimension is layered onto the physical problem— which almost always makes things worse. For example, men often become increasingly anxious that they'll lose their erection. Anxiety releases hormones such as adrenaline that clamp down on blood vessels, including those feeding the penis, thereby making an erection that much harder to obtain. Men sometimes misinterpret the reason for erectile failure

("I must not find her sexually attractive anymore"), and women sometimes blame themselves ("I must not be sexy enough"). The result, as we saw in Norm's case, can be a psychological domino effect leading to less and less sex, and feelings of emotional distance, abandonment, or rejection.

One of my patients, a fifty-year-old man who had recently been remarried to a woman twelve years younger than he, was having erectile problems. His teenage children still lived in the house, which made him feel self-conscious, and he and his new wife both worked long hours, which sapped his energy and sexual performance.

"I just need a little insurance," he told me. "I love my wife and want to make love to her. I just don't want to have to worry about my erection."

This man's situation was a typical combination of the natural age-related decline in performance coupled with some specific lifestyle factors and a fear of failure. For him, the erection-enhancing medication worked beautifully.

"Sometimes I don't even need it," he says. "Over the past few months I've gained enough confidence and feel relaxed enough about sex that sometimes it just happens spontaneously, which is really great."

Not all stories about Viagra end so happily, however. If a couple has become used to not having sex because of erectile problems, it will likely take more than improved erectile function to restore a healthy, mutually satisfying sex life. Harold's story is a good example. Harold was sixty-seven when he came to see me about a prescription for Viagra. He and his wife, Cheryl, hadn't had an active sex life in many years, though he told me they still enjoyed cuddling together in bed and he felt they still loved each other deeply. Harold had read about Viagra and wanted to try it. His symptoms were classic and fairly normal: a slowly diminishing sex drive coupled with erections that were more difficult to obtain and that "wilted" faster than he would have liked.

"I just want to see if these pills really work," Harold told me.

I gave him a trial packet of Viagra, and he left my office with a smile on his face.

A week later Harold called me. He sounded both perplexed and annoyed.

"The pills worked, Doc," he said. "But Cheryl doesn't want to have sex! She was actually angry when I tried to make love to her the other night. I was baffled—and then I got angry back and we had a big fight. She admitted that all this time we weren't having sex was just fine with her and she didn't like me suddenly pushing her to have sex. She said it hurt to have sex now and she just wasn't going to do it."

Harold was understandably frustrated, but as I questioned him more closely, I could see that his approach and behavior were contributing to the problem. He admitted that he hadn't told his wife about the Viagra; he'd wanted it to seem natural. So his wife had undoubtedly been surprised and somewhat confused by his sexual advances. Also, Harold didn't understand how a woman's reproductive organs change with age, so he couldn't appreciate the ways he could help make sex enjoyable. I suggested that Harold be honest with his wife, that he tell her about the Viagra and why he wanted to try it, and that he not push her to have sex if she didn't want it. I also explained that many older women have difficulty becoming sufficiently lubricated for enjoyable sex, so spending a good deal of time on foreplay and using a lubricant of some kind would help.

I'd like to report that Harold did all of this and that he and his wife resolved their differences and discovered that they enjoyed making love with each other. Unfortunately, that didn't happen. I can't say exactly why—I never talked to Harold's wife, for one thing, and I don't know how Harold actually put my advice into practice. What I know is that he called me about ten days later and said he was giving up—that his wife thought he was being juvenile to try Viagra and that nothing he could say would change her mind.

At the end of this chapter I'll talk more about the emotional aspects of sex and ways that couples can avoid this kind of situation. For the moment I just want to reiterate the point that "fixing" an erection is just a small part of solving the much larger puzzle that is any couple's sexual relationship.

The Penis 101

Just as a man will be better prepared to diagnose car problems if he knows how engines work, he will be in a better position

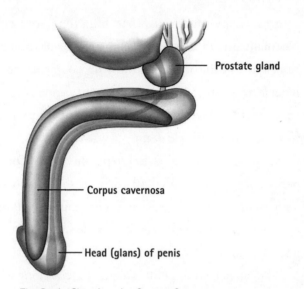

Prostate gland

Corpus cavernosa

Head (glans) of penis

The Penis, Showing the Corpus Cavernosa

to deal effectively with erectile dysfunction if he knows how his penis works.

In most cases, an erection begins when the brain registers a physical or mental stimulation, such as a physical touch or a sexually arousing visual or mental image. This arousal produces electrochemical signals that travel along nerve fibers down the spinal cord to the penis. When the signals reach the penis, they trigger the release of a gas called nitric oxide, which, in turn, causes the arteries feeding the penis to relax and open up. Blood can then pump into two cylinders of spongelike tissue inside the penis—the corpus cavernosa. When the chambers are fully saturated, the penis is erect. The erection is maintained because the swelling tissue squeezes shut the many small veins that drain blood out of the penis. Normally, an erection lasts as long as sexual stimulation continues or until orgasm. Following orgasm, nerve signals reverse the effect on penile arteries, squeezing them shut again, which allows blood to drain out of the penis, causing it to return to the flaccid state.

Erections are actually vital to penile health. Only when the penis is erect is it fully bathed in fresh, oxygen-rich blood. This is why healthy men have numerous spontaneous erections while they sleep; it is their body's way of maintaining a good flow of blood to the tissues of the penis.

The normal adult penis is about 3 inches long when flaccid and between 4.5 and 6.5 inches long when erect. Penises that are longer than average when flaccid tend not to enlarge as much during erection; hence the size of a flaccid penis is not a good indication of its size when erect.

Boys (and men too) tend to be very concerned with the length of their penis, which is probably natural but also can cause much needless anxiety. Male actors in erotic magazines and videos notwithstanding, bigger is not necessarily better when it comes to penis size. Several facts about female anatomy are relevant here. First, vaginas have evolved to accommodate an average-size penis, meaning that much beyond six inches of penis is of little use and may actually cause a woman pain during intercourse when the penis hits her cervix. Second, only the outer third of a woman's vagina is richly endowed with pleasure-producing nerves. The inner two thirds is virtually numb in comparison, hence whether a man's penis reaches to the end of the vagina or not is irrelevant to his ability to satisfy his partner sexually. Finally, the *real* source of a woman's pleasure, the clitoris, isn't in the vagina at all—it's above the mouth of the vagina and usually requires stimulation other than mere penile penetration to produce an orgasm. All of which simply proves the validity of the old saw that "it's not the size of the instrument, it's how you play the tune." Being a good lover has everything to do with personality, technique, and experience and hardly anything to do with the size of the penis.

The nature of the plumbing supporting erections means that anything interrupting the initial opening of the penile arteries (such as cholesterol deposits inside the arteries, damage to the nerves associated with the arteries, or interruption of the nitric oxide signal in the penis) will hurt erections. Likewise, if the penile veins don't close fully, blood can't remain trapped in the penis long enough to sustain an erection. It's here that aging takes its toll—nerve fibers degrade, arteries clog, and the enzymes that create nitric oxide become less robust. It's here, too, that a wide range of prescription medications exert side effects that can interfere with erections. For example, antidepressants belonging to the family of selective serotonin reuptake inhibitors (SSRIs)—of which Prozac is the most familiar—can interfere with both erectile function and the ability to achieve orgasm. In addition, some classes of high blood pressure medications (such as the thiazide diuretics and beta-blockers) also can impair male sexual functioning. Recognizing the role that common prescription medications can play in sexual dysfunction is important because alternative medications are usually available that can produce similar clinical benefits with less risk of sexual problems. If you are taking an antidepressant or beta-blockers and your sex life is affected, talk to your doctor. You might be much happier with a different prescription.

Although erections can fail for many reasons, treatments and interventions are available today to restore erections and reverse this aspect of the male biological clock.

Treating Erectile Dysfunction

In the early 1990s, pharmacologists at the drug company Pfizer were looking for a new drug to treat angina, a type of chest pain associated with constricted coronary blood vessels. They were looking for a compound that would relax those arteries and ease the pain. Animal studies suggested that a molecule dubbed UK-92-480 might work. When the researchers tried it on men, they found that it wasn't terribly effective at easing angina but did have an unusual side effect: many of the men reported getting more frequent and longer-lasting erections. The Pfizer researchers quickly shifted gears, sensing they might have in UK-92-480 the long-sought erection-enhancing pill. At that time, none of the treatments for erectile dysfunction was very natural or convenient, involving injections into the penis of erection-producing compounds, vacuum devices, or surgical implants.

It took years to conduct the necessary clinical trials for safety and effectiveness, but in 1998, UK-92-480, now dubbed Viagra, made its debut. As noted above, it has proven every bit the blockbuster the researchers hoped for.

Viagra works by blocking an enzyme that normally controls the constriction of penile arteries after the release of nitric oxide. With the enzyme blocked, the relaxation triggered by nitric oxide lasts longer and is harder to shut down. The result? Erections that are easier to create and easier to maintain.

As of this writing, three erection-enhancing drugs are available to men in the United States: Viagra, Levitra, and Cialis. All three have been shown in clinical trials to be highly effective. About 80 percent of men say these drugs improve their erections, and about 75 percent of men say they allow them to have intercourse successfully.[1] All three cause the same range of side effects in a minority of men who use them, most commonly headache, facial flushing, runny nose, and stomach upset.

Although all three drugs work the same way (by enhancing the effects of nitric oxide), subtle differences in their molecular shapes result in differences in how long they remain effective in the body.

Viagra and Levitra are typically taken thirty minutes to an hour before sexual activity is expected and maintain their erection-enhancing effects for four to six hours. Cialis has been nicknamed "the weekender" because its effects remain for roughly thirty-six hours, which makes the timing of sexual relations less critical.

It's important to point out that these drugs do not *cause* erections. Nitric oxide must be present in the penis for them to work—and nitric oxide is produced only in response to sexual stimulation (either physical or mental). This is actually something of an advantage because it's more "natural." The earlier treatments involving penile injections produced an "automatic" erection, which some women reported made them feel a bit left out of the sexual process.

It's important to point out, too, that a man has to *want* to get an erection as well as have the *ability* to get an erection. Studies show that Viagra and other erection-enhancing drugs don't work very well in men with low testosterone and, hence, low sexual desire. For these men, testosterone needs to be boosted to normal levels using any of the available strategies (covered fully in Chapter 2), and then, if they still have erectile problems, an erection-enhancing medication is likely to be effective.

It's also vital to remember that all three of these drugs can be dangerous—even lethal—if used by men who are also taking nitrates for heart problems. In addition, if used by otherwise healthy men, the drugs can cause an excessively prolonged and painful erection, called priapism. Fortunately, this is extremely rare. Because of these and other much less common risks, these drugs should always be taken with a doctor's permission.

A summary of the key points about the current erection-enhancing pills is on page 79.

Product	Onset of Action	Duration of Action	Recommended Dose	Not Suitable For	Limits of Use
VIAGRA	30–60 minutes	4 hours	50 mg to start, with adjustments up to 100 mg or down to 25 mg, depending on response	Men taking nitrate medications such as nitroglycerine	Should not be used more than once a day
LEVITRA	25–30 minutes	4–5 hours	10 mg, with adjustment to 20 mg if needed	Men taking nitrate medications or alpha-blocker medications	Should not be used more than once a day
CIALIS	16–60 minutes	Up to 36 hours	10 mg, with adjustment to 20 mg if needed	Men taking nitrate medications or alpha-blocker medications (except Flomax)	Should not be used more than once a day

If Pills Don't Work

Sometimes erectile dysfunction arises from relatively severe damage to either blood vessels or nerves. Older men with diabetes, for instance, often have difficulties with erections because of nerve damage caused by long-term high blood sugar levels. Also, men who have had prostate surgery (even those who undergo so-called nerve-sparing surgery) often have erectile problems because of damage done to nerves during the operation. In such cases, erection-enhancing pills may not be enough. The remaining options include: penile self-injection, intraurethral suppositories, vacuum devices, and penile implants. If a man is found to have abnormally low testosterone levels, he may benefit from testosterone therapy as well (see Chapter 2 for more on this topic).

Injections are made with a short, fine needle into the side of the penile shaft. The injections are virtually painless, although most men wince at the thought of having them. An erection is generally obtained within minutes of the injection and can last from a half hour to an hour. Several drugs are used, including papaverine hydrochloride, phentolamine, and prostaglandins, and a number of different injection systems are available. The main risks of injections are a prolonged, painful erection (priapism) and scarring from repeated use.

An alternate way to deliver the medication is in the form of a tiny pellet deposited about an inch into the penis by inserting an applicator tube into the opening at the tip of the penis. The pellet dissolves, and an erection begins within eight to ten minutes. Discomfort is fairly common, with the most common side effects being aching in the penis, testicles, and the area between the penis and rectum; warmth or a burning sensation in the urethra; redness from increased blood flow to the penis; and minor urethral bleeding or spotting.

Mechanical vacuum devices cause an erection by creating a partial vacuum, which draws blood into the penis, engorging and expanding it. The devices have three components: a plastic cylinder, into which the penis is placed; a pump, which draws air out of the cylinder; and an elastic band, which is placed around the base of the penis to maintain the erection after the cylinder is removed by preventing blood from flowing back into the body.

If none of these methods works and the erectile dysfunction is severe, penile implants can be installed surgically. The most common implants are fluid-filled hydraulic devices that allow a man to have a modest erection any time he wants by pumping fluid into two inflatable chambers implanted in the penis. The disadvantages of implants are their high cost, the discomfort and risks of surgery, and the fact that the erections obtained, while sufficient for intercourse, may not be as robust as those obtained in men with less severe dysfunction who use other methods.

Premature Ejaculation

Sam came to see me about a problem even more common than erectile dysfunction. The number one male sexual problem is premature ejaculation—ejaculation that occurs sooner than desired, either before or shortly after penetration, causing distress to one or both partners. Roughly one in five men between the ages of eighteen and sixty experience premature ejaculation.[2]

Sam had been married for nearly seven years and came to see me only because his wife insisted he see a doctor—a very common pattern. In fact, his wife came with him on the first visit, which I encourage because it's helpful to hear both sides of the story. When I asked Sam if he had a problem with his erections, he said he didn't think so. His wife rolled her eyes.

"Doctor, the thing is that Sam, well, he just doesn't last very long, if you know what I mean," his wife said. "He's in me for maybe thirty seconds—a minute, tops—and he comes and that's it. It's all over before I've even begun, and, I'll tell you, I'm tired of it."

Sam was actually on less of a hair trigger than some men with this problem. Some men are so sensitive that they have an orgasm even before their penis has entered their partner's vagina. Others climax within seconds of entry. It's usually very frustrating for both partners. The man wants much more relaxed, lengthy lovemaking, and the woman, whose orgasmic pattern is naturally longer and slower, never gets the chance to have an orgasm with the man inside her. Doctors need to question men about exactly what they are experiencing because some men don't understand that loss of an erection after ejaculation is normal; thus they wrongly think their problem is erectile dysfunction when the actual problem is premature ejaculation.

Although it's true that premature ejaculation tends to resolve with age—the male biological clock slows down the sexual response cycle—this usually happens long after a great deal of sexual dissatisfaction has already occurred. Fortunately, today premature ejaculation is one of the easiest problems to treat, particularly if a man can talk easily about sex with his partner and they are willing to experiment to find more satisfying ways to have sex.

Although it's common for men who want to slow down their orgasm to try to distract themselves mentally by, for instance, doing math in their heads, this takes the man away from the moment and from a full connection with his partner. A better approach is to begin sexual stimulation until the man feels he is nearing the "point of no return." He either withdraws or the stimulation is discontinued for about thirty seconds. The sequence is repeated as often as needed. In this way the man can gain control and confidence, which may reduce his tension and the associated tendency to ejaculate prematurely.

A variation of this method is to gently squeeze the penis where the glans meets the penile shaft during the "break" periods just described. Some men report that this reduces their urge to ejaculate.

In recent years doctors have seized on a normally undesirable side effect of some antidepressants to help men with premature ejaculation. The class of antidepressants called selective serotonin reuptake inhibitors inhibit orgasm in many of the men who take them. Prozac was the first antidepressant in this class, but Zoloft, Paxil, and Luvox are also members. A member of the older class of tricyclic antidepressants, Anafranil, is also sometimes prescribed. Low doses of such drugs have proven very helpful for men suffering from premature ejaculation.[3] Effective doses range from about half the normal daily dose to doses typically used in depressed patients. Although the antidepressant effects of SSRIs typically take several weeks to kick in, their orgasm-delaying effects happen within about four hours, which means that men can use them periodically if they want.

Many men, however, prefer to simply take one pill a day so they don't have to think about it and can respond to romantic situations more spontaneously.

Some men use one of a variety of anesthetic creams that numb the penis mildly and so delay orgasm. The creams must be used carefully, since using too much can cause an erection to fail from lack of sensation. If used without a condom, the cream may also cause vaginal numbness in the partner. Condoms alone can reduce penile sensation sufficiently in some men with premature ejaculation to have satisfactory sex.

I gave Sam a prescription for a low dose of Zoloft. A week later he called and said that things had definitely improved, but his wife thought he should try a higher dose. I raised the dose to that normally used by people who are depressed.

"It's unbelievable," Sam said two weeks later. "For the first time in my life I've actually made love for fifteen or twenty minutes. My wife and I even had simultaneous orgasms the other night—and *that's* never happened before, believe me!"

Like most men, Sam felt some minor side effects in the first week of taking the medication—slight stomach queasiness and a mild headache. Both have now disappeared.

"It's kind of a double-whammy effect," Sam says. "I'm happier because I can finally have good sex with my wife, and maybe I'm a little happier because of the antidepressant. Whatever—it's great."

The advent of safe, effective pills to enhance erectile function and, in effect, reverse this aspect of the male biological clock has been a tremendous boon to both men and their partners. But as we saw with Harold's story, an erection is hardly the whole story of sex. When an erection-enhancing pill actually makes a relationship *worse,* the problem is often the man's lack of appreciation that real intimacy is about more than mechanics, erections, penetration, and orgasm. Most women enjoy sex, but not if intimacy is absent. Many things contribute to romantic intimacy between people, of course, but some key factors are honesty, good communication, mutual respect, emotional security, healthy self-esteem, and a good body image. All of these can take years to develop, and if they've disappeared in a relationship (or if they never existed in the first place) no amount of soft music, candles, sexy underwear, or Viagra is going to do the trick.

I often joke with the partners of my male patients that if I could invent a listening pill—a pill that would make men pay attention to women and simply listen without interrupting— I'd be a billionaire. Since that's not going to happen, I simply want to pass on this advice to men:

- Include your partner in your decision to explore erection-enhancing pills or techniques.
- Listen to your partner; let her talk.
- Don't interrupt.
- Pay attention to your partner's emotional, as well as physical, desires.
- In lovemaking, relax and go slowly—at least at first.

When a couple can talk openly about sex, when they approach a problem such as erectile dysfunction as a team, when they avoid casting blame, and when they have an experimental or playful approach to trying new things, the chances are very, very good that they will both be far more satisfied with sex than they were before. One last thing: women, particularly postmenopausal women, can have sexual dysfunction just as men do and may also need assistance with desire or arousal. Such problems as painful sex, inability to achieve orgasm, thinning of vaginal tissues, lack of sexual desire, and inability to lubricate can seriously affect a couple's sex life. Since this is a book about male sexual function, a complete discussion of the many treatment approaches to female sexual dysfunction is not included. But women should know that many options exist, including the use of vibrators to enhance orgasm, different sexual positions to minimize pain, relaxation techniques, vaginal exercises, and more pharmacological approaches such as estrogen creams or testosterone replacement therapy.

4

Infertility: Not Just a Woman's Problem

Robbing a man of his fertility is the most wrenching potential effect of the male biological clock. Although not as common as age-related sexual performance problems, male infertility remains a huge problem. Infertility is usually defined as an inability to conceive after a year of unprotected sex, but that's not carved in stone. These days, I find that many older couples do not want to wait that long and seek help much sooner.

An estimated one of every ten men trying to conceive a child—roughly 2.5 million men in the United States alone—are either infertile or subfertile. Many of these men don't know they have a problem because they haven't been tested, while others have been tested but not thoroughly enough. Hence their problem remains undetected and medical attention is focused on the woman. (Recall that in about 40 percent of infertile couples it's the man who has the problem, in another 40 percent it's the woman, and in the last 20 percent either both partners contribute or the cause is unknown.)

In this chapter I'll review the most common problems with male fertility and how to fix them without resorting to *in vitro* fertilization (IVF). Again, I'm not against the appropriate use of IVF. But I do believe that the widespread availability of IVF and the profit motive of the clinics offering these services are leading to couples' being steered to IVF *before* the man has been thoroughly examined and *before* much less expensive and demanding treatment options have been explored. (Chapter 5 examines IVF in detail.)

Several recent studies have looked at the relative costs of fixing various types of male infertility problems without IVF versus the cost of "treating" male infertility with IVF.[1] The results are striking and are summed up in the graph on the next page.

The light-colored bars show the cost of successfully treating four of the most common causes of male infertility (I'll discuss these in a minute). The cost averages around $20,000 per successful delivery of a baby. The dark gray bars show the cost of "treating" these four conditions with IVF—specifically, a combination of *in vitro* fertilization with a technique for inserting sperm directly into a woman's egg (intracytoplasmic sperm injection (ICSI) is covered in Chapter 5). These procedures cost anywhere from $60,000 to $80,000 per delivery, reflecting the fact that, on average, most couples must go through multiple cycles of IVF to achieve pregnancy and delivery.

The Cost of a Single Birth: Male Treatments Versus
IVF-Intracytoplasmic Sperm Injection

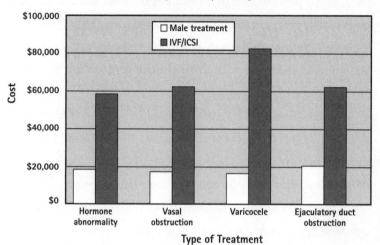

Ironically, some states and some health insurance companies now pay for IVF services but *not* for "low-tech" treatments of specific causes of male infertility. This is another reason that couples often move ahead with IVF before they should. I'm not against health coverage of infertility treatments, but I believe that any insurance company or government agency that professes concern for "family values" is obliged to help cover the costs of creating those families in the first place. If some types of infertility treatment are covered, *all* treatments should be covered, particularly the less expensive, less invasive treatments for male infertility.

But cost isn't the only reason men and women should thoroughly explore the non-IVF options for treating male infertility. As we'll see in the next chapter, these technologies place significant logistical and physical burdens on a couple, particularly the woman. Failing to check adequately for problems on the male side and failing to try fixing male-factor problems first, results in unfairly shifting the burden for "correcting" a couple's infertility to the woman.

Finally, although IVF technologies have improved greatly over the years, they unavoidably short-circuit an important part of natural conception. A woman's reproductive tract poses a natural obstacle course for sperm deposited in the vagina during unprotected sex. Only the strongest sperm can reach an egg—and as we've seen, the health of a sperm cell is correlated with the quality of the genetic information that it contains. This "survival of the fittest" aspect of natural intercourse is nature's way of weeding out sperm that might contain genetic malfunctions.

IVF technologies, however, must often be done with sperm obtained directly from a testicle or other part of the male reproductive tract, or from ejaculate that has been treated to help the sperm survive. As good as the current IVF procedures are, the rate of congenital abnormalities among babies born via IVF is double that of babies conceived naturally— 9 percent versus 4.2 percent.[2] This, of course, is not an ideal situation, but most couples accept this risk if IVF is their only choice for having a baby. Yet many couples do have a choice— they need to try to fix treatable problems in the male partner *before* jumping to IVF.

Diagnosing Infertility

As we've seen, at practically every stage of the male biological clock, things can go wrong in ways that affect fertility. But it usually takes some medical detective work to figure out what exactly is malfunctioning in any one man. Sometimes the problem is apparent as soon as a man drops his shorts for a physical examination of his genitals. For example, the distended blood vessels of a varicocele are usually easy to spot—at least for physicians who are trained to look for them and appreciate their importance. But most other problems take more time, and sometimes, despite our best efforts, the cause is never found.

It's important to remember, however, that even when tests fail to find the exact cause, infertility is *always* a sign of a medical condition, not a psychological or personal problem.

One of the most critical steps in diagnosing a reproductive problem is often the least appreciated—by both patients and doctors. A careful medical history is the foundation on which all further tests and examinations rest. This means asking a lot of very specific questions about aspects of a man's body and behavior that are typically very private, such as how often a man masturbates and how, exactly, the semen spurts out of the penis at orgasm. These are important questions, and the answers may hold clues to what is going wrong, so it's important to be as straightforward and honest as possible when answering. Here are some of the questions typically asked during an infertility workup:

- Have you ever caused a conception with another partner?
- How long have you been having unprotected sex with your current partner?
- Do you use any lubricants during sex?
- Have you been timing sex to get pregnant, and, if so, what methods have you been using?
- Do any physical or sexual problems interfere with effective intercourse?
- Do you smoke or use any recreational drugs (including alcohol)?
- Do you know of any fertility problems in any immediate blood relatives?

A doctor will also ask detailed questions about any prescription medications a man currently uses, as well as his history of disease, accidents, and hospitalizations (if any). The physician will also ask about conditions in the workplace and home to check for the possibility that pollutants may be contributing to the problem.

After taking a detailed medical history, the physician should conduct a physical examination, paying particular attention to the genitals. The penis and testicles will be carefully and gently examined for any abnormalities. In general, testicles are about the size of walnuts and have a firm, smooth, rubbery feel. Undersized testicles (the size of cherries or smaller) can be a sign of low sperm counts, low testosterone levels, or, as we saw in Chapter 2, unusually high testosterone levels resulting from testosterone replacement. Small testicles are usually a sign of impaired fertility.

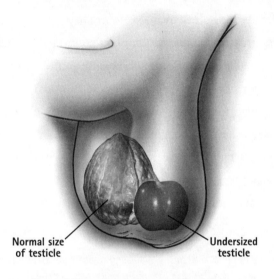

Normal size
of testicle

Undersized
testicle

Sizes of Normal and Abnormal Testicles

The testicles will also be checked for abnormalities such as varicoceles, tumors, or fluid-filled cysts called hydroceles. The penis will be checked to make sure that the urethral opening is at the tip of the penis and that the foreskin of an uncircumcised man can retract easily.

Many men these days are not given proper or thorough physical examinations by their doctors. I know this because I pick up many more cases of testicular cancer, varicoceles, and other testicular problems than are reported to be average among doctors. That's because I do a very thorough job, not just a cursory examination. I'm not suggesting that I'm the only doctor doing correct examinations, but clearly other doctors, most of whom are probably *not* urologists, are not specifically trained to evaluate infertility.

The prostate gland, which plays a vital role in ejaculation, is examined with a digital rectal exam or ultrasound.

The prostate, you will recall, secretes much of the fluid in semen during orgasm. It sits against the rear wall of the rectum, so its shape, size, and degree of firmness can be felt by a doctor who inserts a gloved finger into the rectum. This isn't a particularly enjoyable process for most men, but it's not painful and it is essential to getting a complete picture of a man's reproductive

Side View of the Rectum, Bladder, Prostate, Penis, and Scrotum, Showing the Position of the Prostate Against the Rectal Wall

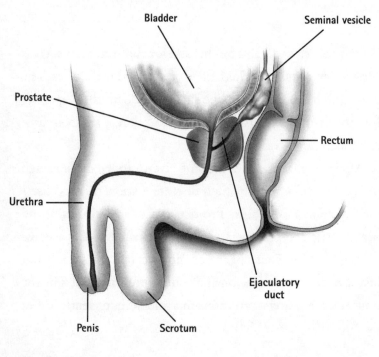

machinery. (It might help to remember that women are subjected to similar types of invasive physical exams starting at a far younger age and on a more regular basis than are men.)

The final step in the basic examination is a thorough semen analysis, the details of which I discussed in Chapter 1. Remember that a simple sperm count is not enough. The vigor with which the sperm swim (motility) must be measured, the shape of the sperm (morphology) must be assessed, and various other aspects of the seminal fluid must be analyzed, such as the amount of fluid and the time it takes for the semen to liquefy after being ejaculated.

An often overlooked step in a good semen analysis is a check for infection in the reproductive tract. This is best done two ways: by counting white cells in the semen and by culturing a sample of semen to see if bacteria are present. White cells are part of the body's defense against invaders; hence a high level of white cells in semen is a sign of an infection or sexually transmitted disease, both of which can hurt fertility. Culturing semen involves spreading a sample on a substance conducive to bacterial growth (a growth medium) and incubating it for several days to see if bacteria are present. Many urologists do not order semen cultures because they claim that they are always contaminated with germs from the skin, but two recent studies have proven them wrong.[3] As long as a man has washed his hands and genitals and catches his ejaculate in a sterile container, a semen culture is a reliable indicator of an infection.

A summary of the various normal measures of semen we've discussed thus far is on the next page.

Normal Semen Values

Volume	2–5 milliliters (ml) or more
Sperm concentration (often called the sperm "count")	20 million per ml or more
Percentage of active sperm (often called "motility")	50 percent or more
Morphology (strict)	14 percent or more of sperm observed should have normal shape
Viscosity after liquefaction	3 or less on a 0–4 scale in which 0 is extremely liquid and runny, and 4 is thick and gel-like
White cells (sometimes called "round cells")	1 million cells per ml or less

If below-normal results are found on any part of a semen analysis, a second test is usually performed within a week or two to confirm the results. Many things can affect the results of a semen analysis, such as how often a man has sex and whether a man has lately had even a minor illness, such as a cold or the flu, associated with a fever. You should never proceed with any type of treatment for infertility based only on a single abnormal semen analysis!

Any abnormal test results may lead the doctor to order further tests to get to the root of the problem. For example, if a man's semen does not liquefy quickly or completely, his doctor may order a test that will detect the presence of antibodies in the sperm. Research suggests that some men's immune systems treat sperm as foreign invaders. The immune system creates antibodies (special molecules in the blood and other bodily fluids that "tag" a foreign substance for destruction) against a man's sperm. These antibodies coat the sperm, which can cause them to clump together or react badly to the mucus and fluids in a woman's reproductive tract. Antisperm antibodies may also interfere with penetration and fertilization of eggs. Three types of antisperm antibodies have been detected, and tests can reveal if they are present in a man's semen. If so, some techniques have been developed for rapidly washing the sperm to reduce the number that have antibodies attached to them. The washed sperm can then be injected into a woman's uterus, a process called intrauterine insemination (IUI), described more fully later in this chapter.

Another test that is sometimes conducted is called a "sperm penetration assay," also known as a "hamster egg test." This evaluates the sperm's ability to break through the outer membrane of a hamster egg and fuse with the egg cytoplasm, which is a critical step in fertilization. (The hamster eggs are treated to make them good models for human eggs. Fertilization cannot occur because the species are so different.) A test used less commonly these days is the cervical mucus penetration test, which uses cow mucus to simulate a woman's cervical mucus, through which sperm must swim to get to the uterus and fallopian tubes. If sperm can't get through these substances, their motility is weak and some form of assisted technology, such as IUI or IVF, is usually recommended.

If a blockage is suspected in some part of a man's reproductive tract, ultrasound can be used to try to pinpoint the problem. To see structures in the testicles, an ultrasound wand can be moved over the skin of the scrotum. The best way to see the seminal vesicles, vas deferens, and prostate gland is to use a special lubricated ultrasound wand that is passed into the rectum. It's a fast, painless procedure and can be essential in diagnosing easily correctable problems such as blocked ejaculatory ducts.

If no sperm are found in a man's semen, several kinds of tests may be ordered to pinpoint the problem. The simplest one looks for a sugar called fructose in the semen. Fructose, which is common in fruits, is made in the human body only in the seminal vesicles and vas deferens; therefore, if the test finds no fructose in the semen, the vesicles and vas deferens may be blocked or absent because of a congenital defect.

Tests that determine if the testicles are making sperm involve a testicular biopsy. Three types of biopsies can be done: fine-needle aspiration, needle biopsy, and open biopsy. Biopsy using any of these methods usually doesn't require a hospital stay, and recovery is typically rapid and only mildly uncomfortable.

Fine-needle aspiration is the most minor procedure and is used to confirm if mature sperm cells are present in a testis. The scrotum is numbed with a local anesthetic, a thin hypodermic needle is inserted, and a small amount of testicular tissue is withdrawn. The tissue (called the aspirate) is quickly analyzed for the presence and quality of sperm.

Needle biopsy uses a larger-diameter needle that removes a small core of tissue. Its advantage is that more tissue is removed, giving a greater chance of finding sperm. Again, a local anesthetic is used and the degree of discomfort is mild.

Open biopsy involves making an opening in the skin of the scrotum, revealing a testis or other structure for examination, and removing a small slice of tissue using special surgical scissors. The opening is usually closed with a few stitches, and the man is asked to hold ice on the area for the first day to reduce swelling, and he is told to avoid vigorous activity for a few days.

Whether or not any of these extra tests is done, both men and their partners should carefully read the results of the semen analysis and any other tests done and ask the doctor to clarify any confusing points. Doctors are often busy and, without meaning to, may rush through an explanation of the results or use unfamiliar words or phrases. Don't be afraid to interrupt and ask for an explanation! Most doctors appreciate patients who want to understand the details of their diagnosis and treatment.

Pinpointing the cause of a problem in the male reproductive system is not usually a complicated, expensive, or arduous process. But that doesn't mean a cause is always found; sometimes we just don't know why a man has no sperm in his semen, for example. But by and large, an answer is found, and usually relatively quickly. The real challenge in diagnosing male infertility is simply getting a man into the office for the analysis in the first place and finding a doctor who is thoroughly familiar with male infertility. (See the appendix for help in locating a qualified local urologist.)

Fixing Male Infertility Problems

Common sense suggests that when dealing with a fertility problem, a man try the simplest, least expensive methods first. That means, for example, taking an antibiotic to clear up a suspected infection or using a medication such as Clomid to boost sperm production rather than immediately jumping to assisted reproduction such as IVF. Unfortunately, some doctors dismiss such relatively easy steps, either out of ignorance or out of a desire to give their patients some tangible results as quickly as possible.

Here I'll review the most common male infertility problems and discuss how to treat them. I'm going to emphasize treatments that do *not* rely on IVF or other techniques that involve manipulating both egg and sperm. As I've already mentioned, I've seen too many couples who neglect to consider these relatively low-tech approaches and rush right into the expensive and complicated arena of assisted reproductive technologies such as IVF.

Infections

One of the most underappreciated causes of impaired male fertility is an infection in some part of the reproductive tract, most commonly the prostate gland, seminal vesicles, or epididymis. (See Chapter 1 for a comprehensive discussion of the male reproductive anatomy.) Such infections are often subclinical, meaning they don't produce noticeable symptoms, but the waste products produced by the bacteria can change the chemical conditions in these structures in ways that damage or kill sperm.

In addition, the irritation to surrounding tissues can cause swelling or an immune response that can impair sperm function or movement. Infections should always be ruled out as a factor in infertility because they are so easy and inexpensively treated. (Note that if an infection is found in the man, *both* partners need to be treated with antibiotics to ensure that the woman doesn't reinfect the man.) I have seen many cases of men with subclinical infections who got their partners pregnant after years of trying once their infections were cleared up with antibiotic treatment.

The incidence of reproductive tract infections clearly increases the longer the biological clock ticks. The largest study done to date on the subject found that about 6 percent of men had such an infection but that more than twice as many men over forty had an infection.[4] This story of one of my patients illustrates this issue.

Todd is a staff physician in a thriving urban infertility and IVF clinic. With two children of his own, both conceived naturally within a normal amount of time spent trying, Todd didn't think he'd ever be in the position of the couples he saw every day in his practice. But as Todd and his wife tried for a third child, nothing happened. A year passed, then another.

"I was evaluated, my wife was evaluated—they didn't find anything," Todd says. "I was thirty-five at the time and my wife was thirty-three, so we thought, 'Okay, we're both getting older, maybe that's what's going on.'"

Todd and his wife were reluctantly beginning to think about using assisted reproductive techniques when he called me up to ask what I thought. From what he told me, I suspected a low-grade infection. An ultrasound examination at my office showed that his prostate had some areas of scar tissue usually seen when a man has had a prior infection. A healthy prostate is a perfect breeding ground for bacteria because of its spongelike structure, which is riddled with small, crooked passageways. Todd gave a semen sample that was sent out for culturing. In a few days my hunch was confirmed: his semen contained enterococcus bacteria, which are a common cause of urinary tract infections but are difficult to kill with most antibiotics when located in the prostate.

I put Todd and his wife on a strong antibiotic for four weeks, during which time he and his wife continued to have sex. A month after the course of antibiotic was finished, Todd phoned with happy news: his wife was pregnant.

"I was pleasantly surprised that that's all it took," Todd says. "My wife and I weren't terribly thrilled with the idea of going through *in vitro* fertilization. Taking an antibiotic is just such an easy thing to do before getting involved in the high-tech therapies."

Todd's case is hardly unique. The incidence of infection-related infertility is relatively high, though the true scope of the problem is hard to pin down because, as with Todd, many men don't even know they have an infection until a test shows it. As noted previously, studies show that the incidence of infection of the male reproductive tract rises steadily with age.

The epididymis, seminal vesicles, and vas deferens can also be affected—and again, such infections often produce no symptoms. (Acute infections, of course, produce fever and often severe pain, so such cases are seldom ignored.)

Fortunately, even though it can be unusually difficult to wipe out a reproductive tract infection, total annihilation isn't always necessary. In Todd's case, for example, a semen sample cultured several months after he had stopped taking the antibiotic still contained some bacteria, but the infection had clearly been knocked down enough to open a window of opportunity for conception.

Clogged Ejaculatory Ducts

Sometimes untreated infection, physical injury, or surgery partially or completely blocks the tiny slitlike holes through which sperm are propelled into the prostate during orgasm.

Blocked ejaculatory ducts, however, are not always obvious, which was the case for George. From time to time, George noticed that his semen was tinged pink with blood. The discovery was too uncomfortable for him to talk about, even to his wife.

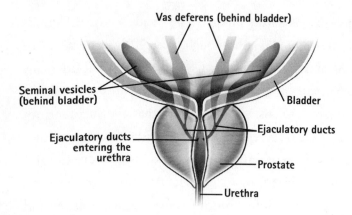

Close-up View of the Prostate showing the Ejaculatory Ducts

"You feel embarrassed," he says. "You don't just go tell someone, 'Hey, I got blood in my semen.'"

He finally confided in a buddy, who urged him to get checked out by a urologist. When George's wife, Shawna, found out about it, she pressed him too.

George and Shawna had been diagnosed with "unexplained infertility" four years earlier, when they had been trying to have their first child. At the time George was evaluated and found that his sperm count, while on the low side, was still in the range considered normal. Shawna, meanwhile, underwent a host of diagnostic tests, including surgical examination of her ovaries. Doctors found nothing during the procedure, so the couple embarked on the process of IUI combined with regular hormone shots to stimulate ovulation.

Unfortunately, Shawna experienced a serious side effect from the hormones.

"I had cysts form on my ovaries," she says. "They were afraid that if I kept going with the injections the cysts would get bigger, so twice I stopped the treatments."

Finally she ovulated, and some of George's semen was injected into her uterus. Nine months later their first son was born.

"It was so frustrating while we were trying," Shawna says. "Because all our friends were pregnant or had kids, and every time we went out people would say, 'So when are you having a kid?' I was very emotional. We really wanted to have a child, and so we were very, very happy when Lester arrived."

Now, four years later, they wanted another baby, and George's pink semen didn't bode well for their chances. It was hard enough looking ahead to another time-consuming and potentially risky round of IUI.

What they didn't know was that they didn't need IUI to get pregnant—and most likely hadn't needed it to conceive Lester. Like many other couples, George and Shawna were victims of the bias against looking carefully at the male in cases of infertility. If the doctors had done more thorough tests on George, they probably would have found what I did: George's ejaculatory ducts were clogged because of a low-grade bacterial infection that had been present for years. I suspected this when I took a careful medical history and George reported that in the past few years he seemed to be ejaculating less and less semen at orgasm and that the semen dribbled out of his penis instead of spurting out.

If the ejaculatory ducts are completely closed, a man is sterile. If the ducts are partially clogged, his sperm count will be low, reducing (but not eliminating) his fertility.

The blood in George's semen—a condition called "hemato-spermia"—was a clear sign of a prostate infection. A semen culture confirmed George's diagnosis, and like most men he was surprised by the diagnosis because he had no fever, pain, or burning sensation during urination.

George's infection had been so chronic that his ejaculatory ducts were scarred and partially clogged. Using a rectal ultra-sound probe, I could clearly see the scarring on the ejacula-tory ducts as well as significant enlargement of his seminal vesicles. His seminal vesicles, which provide roughly 60 per-cent of semen volume, were backing up with seminal fluids because they couldn't empty properly during ejaculation. The semen dripped out rather than shot out.

The standard treatment for blocked ejaculatory ducts is transurethral resection of the ejaculatory ducts, or TURED. "Transurethral" means "through the urethra." In this case, it means that a thin tube called a cystoscope is passed through the opening at the tip of the penis and guided up to the center of the prostate, where the ejaculatory ducts are located. The cysto-scope is equipped with a lens that allows the doctor to see exactly where the ducts are in the urethra. "Resection" means "removal of tissue." When the cystoscope is positioned cor-rectly, a tiny shaver is manipulated by the doctor and a thin

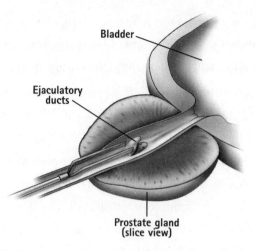

Transurethral Resection of the Ejaculatory Ducts (TURED)

layer, or "chip," of the scarred tissue is removed from the ejaculatory ducts, effectively opening them completely. Fortunately, very little blood usually flows during this procedure, so the ducts, which are tiny, do not become reclogged with blood clots.

When I explained all of this to George, he had the typical male reaction: "Are you kidding me?" he asked. Most men don't like the idea of undergoing any kind of procedure that affects their penis or testicles, and the whole field of transurethral surgery is understandably unfamiliar. But as soon as I explained that there would be no lasting pain, that fertility would improve, and his orgasms were likely to be more prolonged and pleasurable after the procedure, George was willing to move forward with the surgery.

The TURED procedure takes about an hour. Either general anesthesia or spinal anesthesia can be used, depending on the patient and the doctor. After the surgery a thin tube called a catheter is passed into the bladder through the urethra to allow urination while the surgical site heals. The catheter is removed after one or two hours. The penis and general area around and behind the penis are sore for a couple of days. The man should refrain from ejaculating for a week to ten days. The first few ejaculations may contain some blood, but semen color and quality usually return to normal quickly.

It's a relatively simple operation, but, like any surgery, it demands practice and experience in order to avoid complications or inadvertent damage. Men and their partners should make sure they go to a board-certified urologist who has performed this operation in the past. Ask for recommendations from your general physician or friends, and don't be afraid to ask questions when consulting with the urologist.

The TURED, along with the antibiotics to clear up the infection, were all that George needed. His ejaculatory volume increased significantly, to about 4.5 cubic centimeters, and his sperm count and sperm motility became normal. He also reported that his orgasms were much stronger and more satisfying. Two months later, Shawna was pregnant with their daughter, Tonya, and then, eight months after Tonya's birth, she became pregnant with their third child, Charles.

"It's a little uncomfortable for a few days after the procedure, and nobody really likes to give semen samples, but I'm glad I had it done," George says. "I've got three beautiful kids and feel very lucky."

Shawna concurs. "I'm just so happy we went to see Dr. Fisch and that he knew what to look for before we started on the fertility drugs and IVF the second time," she says.

Varicoceles

A varicocele is a bundle of enlarged veins in the scrotum that feels like a bag of worms and is caused by defects in the tiny valves inside the veins. Because the valves don't close properly, blood pools in the veins and warms the testes unnaturally. This interferes with the temperature-sensitive cells that make sperm. Many men don't realize they have a varicocele because the veins typically don't hurt and don't change the quality of their orgasm or ejaculation.

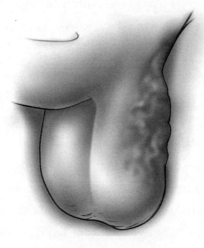

Scrotum with Varicocele

Varicoceles are relatively common, occurring in roughly 20 percent of the male population in general, though that figure masks a definite effect of aging because it averages the percentage across all ages when, in fact, the incidence of varicoceles rises with age. Several studies show that varicoceles are strongly associated with infertility and that they cause a progressive erosion in the quality of sperm over time.[5] Because varicoceles get worse with time, it's vitally important that doctors look for them starting in adolescence, when they first tend to form. Untreated adolescent varicoceles can result in undersized testicles, lower semen volumes, lower sperm counts, and more misshapen sperm.[6]

I believe that many early-stage varicoceles are currently going undetected and that, as they get worse, they impair male fertility in later years. Many doctors still don't recognize the role that varicoceles play in male infertility and may minimize the importance of having a varicocele corrected surgically. This attitude is changing slowly, but if you or your partner encounter skepticism about or resistance to getting a varicocele treated, I suggest you look for another urologist. The following case from my practice illustrates some of the points about varicoceles I've just been discussing.

Michael and Cheryl had been married for two years and decided to start trying to have a child on a cruise to Bermuda. After six months, they began to get worried but figured it might have something to do with the fact that they both were nearing forty.

"We both work incredible hours and have very high-stress

jobs," Cheryl says. "We were buying a house, and we thought those were all contributing factors. We just never slowed down."

Several months later Michael went to a local urologist, who did a basic semen analysis and physical exam.

"He said my sperm count was on the low side of normal and that he saw a small varicocele but that it wasn't anything to worry about," Michael says.

Meanwhile Cheryl had a complete fertility workup, including a laparoscopic surgical examination of her ovaries.

"They found nothing," Cheryl says. "I was shocked because ten years earlier I had to have my left ovary out because of a dermoid cyst, and I was thinking all this time that maybe I had scar tissue or something. But they said everything with me was perfectly healthy."

When Michael and Cheryl finally came to see me, they were frustrated by the lack of answers and by the reluctance on the part of their doctors to consider seriously what I felt were two important findings: I believed the varicocele was much more severe than Michael's doctor did, and when I did a semen culture I also found signs of a urinary tract infection. I recommended that both undergo a course of antibiotics and that the varicocele be repaired as quickly as possible.

"My gynecologist didn't see the importance of Michael having that surgery, first of all, and treating us with antibiotics, secondly," says Cheryl. "He said, 'Oh, that's not important.' I was really frustrated."

When I operated on Michael, I found a set of very large veins—much larger than I had suspected. The surgery itself is relatively simple, and a man is usually up and around the next day. But because it takes three months for new sperm to form and mature, we wouldn't know if getting rid of the varicocele had any effect until autumn. In the meantime, because the infection still hadn't cleared, I kept them on antibiotics. (Fairly often an initial course of antibiotics won't clear a stubborn infection, so couples should always be rechecked after they finish their antibiotics.)

"It was Halloween and we were walking around with our nephews and nieces, out on the sidewalk, and Dr. Fisch called me on my cell phone with my test results," Michael says. "It was kind of a funny place to be talking about my sperm count, you know? But he said everything looked great, the sperm looked good, and the infection was gone. I turned to Cheryl and said, 'Hon, we can go for it.' I was elated."

Michael and Cheryl believe they conceived that Christmas Eve. Two weeks after that, Cheryl did a pregnancy test that came up positive. The following September, after a normal pregnancy, their son, Colin, was born, weighing 8.9 pounds.

Correcting Varicoceles

Surgery to correct varicoceles involves locating the distended veins and tying them off or blocking them in some way to prevent blood from pooling in them. There are three main surgical techniques used to correct a varicocele and one nonsurgical technique. Which method is best depends on the particulars of a man's anatomy, the nature and location of the varicocele, whether previous surgery has been performed, and other factors such as the surgeon's preference and/or amount of experience. Some techniques, such as the one I used on Michael, are done microsurgically with only minimal anesthetic, which shortens the recovery time and poses less risk. As with most microsurgery, practice makes perfect, so be sure to choose a urologic microsurgeon with demonstrated expertise in these techniques.

Varicocele surgery is usually done on an outpatient basis. Most men stay home from work for two or three days. They shouldn't lift anything heavy or exercise strenuously for two weeks. The results of varicocele repairs in thousands of men show an overall improvement in semen quality of about 60 to 70 percent and an overall pregnancy rate of about 40 percent without the need for assisted reproductive technology.

Vasectomy Reversal

Vasectomy is the intentional cutting of the vas deferens to prevent pregnancy. Although only about 1 percent of men who have had a vasectomy later decide that they would like to have children, that translates into about five thousand men each year in the United States alone who want a reversal. Fortunately, the advent of advanced microsurgical techniques and equipment has made vasectomy reversal both common and successful. Repairing a vasectomy is extremely delicate surgery, but with the proper tools in the hands of an experi-

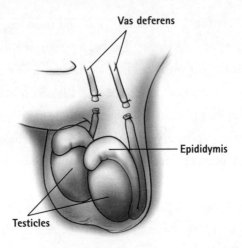

Vas deferens

Epididymis

Testicles

Vasectomy

enced and skilled surgeon, the success rate for vasectomy reversal ranges from 65 to 97 percent.

Two basic types of vasectomy reversal may be performed, depending on the location of the original cuts and how much of the vas deferens remains intact. The most common form, called a "vasovasostomy," stitches the cut ends of the vas deferens together. If the vas must be attached directly to the epididymis, the surgery is called a "vasoepididymostomy."

Recent studies show a success rate of 85 to 97 percent of men undergoing a vasovasostomy, with about half of those couples subsequently achieving a pregnancy. The success rate for vasoepididymostomy is somewhat lower: about 65 percent of men, with approximately 20 percent of the couples subsequently achieving a pregnancy. In either case, the longer it's been since the original vasectomy, the lower the chances for a successful reversal.

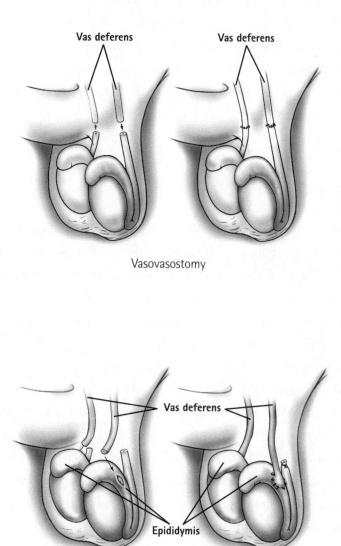

Vas deferens

Vas deferens

Vasovasostomy

Vas deferens

Epididymis

Vasoepididymostomy

Again, training, practice, and skill make a big difference in the success rates of different surgeons. Vasectomy reversal is very exacting because the inner diameter of the vas deferens is barely perceptible to the naked eye and the suture threads are finer than a human hair. Even with the latest operating microscopes, the surgery is extremely delicate.

Vasectomy reversals are usually done on an outpatient basis using local, regional, or general anesthesia, depending on the preference of the surgeon and patient. General anesthesia is often used because it's more comfortable for a patient, given that a vasovasostomy averages two to three hours and a vasoepididymostomy may take as long as four hours. The degree of discomfort after vasectomy reversal varies from patient to patient. The pain is usually similar to or slightly more severe than that of the original vasectomy.

It takes up to six months for sperm counts, motility, and other sperm characteristics to return to prevasectomy levels. The average time from reversal surgery to conception is twelve months. Most pregnancies occur within twenty-four months of reversal surgery.

For reasons that remain unknown, some men who have an initially successful reversal and good sperm counts and motility show a decline in their sperm count and quality after a year or two. Because of this, some doctors recommend that men bank their sperm for later use if needed, particularly after a vasoepididymostomy.

Although it is not technically a "reversal," men who have

had a vasectomy can often have children using a technique to retrieve sperm directly from their testicle or epididymis, coupled with *in vitro* fertilization. (See Chapter 5 for a detailed discussion of this procedure.)

Even though reversal surgery these days is usually successful, some doctors, including myself, routinely do a sperm retrieval at the time of the reversal surgery. The sperm are then frozen so that in the unlikely event the reversal fails, the man can still try to have a child using IVF.

Ejaculation Problems

A variety of relatively uncommon conditions can cause a man's semen to go the wrong way in the urethra during orgasm—meaning up into the bladder instead of out through the penis. Called retrograde ejaculation, this condition can be caused by prostate surgery, bladder surgery, diabetes, or certain medications (such as certain drugs to treat high blood pressure) that prevent the bladder neck from closing tightly during orgasm. Men with spinal cord injuries may also have retrograde ejaculation. As with other problems with male sexuality, the incidence of ejaculation problems increases with advancing age.

If retrograde ejaculation is a side effect of a medication, switching medications or lowering the dose may allow normal ejaculation to occur. For example, one study found that between 5 and 14 percent of men taking Flomax (tamsulosin), a drug to ease urination, experienced retrograde ejaculation but that the incidence was lower with the more selective drug Uroxatral (alfuzosin). If the cause is related to an injury or surgical side effect, assisted reproductive technology using sperm extracted from the bladder, epididymis, or testis can be used, usually with good results since sperm quality and quantity are usually unaffected by this condition.

Undescended Testicles

The testes of a male fetus lie in his abdomen for the first seven months of development. Then, around two months before birth, the testes begin to drop from the abdomen down to the scrotum, dragging their supplying blood vessels and nerves along behind them. In roughly 1 percent of boys, however, one or both testicles fail to descend from the abdomen, a condition called cryptorchidism. If the testes do not descend by the child's first birthday, the condition should be corrected surgically. If the surgery is successful and done early enough, fertility should not be seriously impaired, but sometimes as a boy ages, the effects of early cryptorchidism become more apparent and fertility is reduced. If the condition is not corrected, or is corrected too many years after birth, the testes will not produce sperm.

Injury

As most men know from painful personal experience, the testicles are vulnerable to all manner of physical injury. Sometimes such injury causes scars to form in the epididymis or vas deferens that block sperm movement. Other times the nerves or blood supply to the testicles is disrupted, which can also reduce fertility. Finally, sometimes the vas deferens or testicles are injured accidentally in the course of surgery, such as that to repair a hernia or correct an undescended testicle. Blockages caused by scar tissue can often be either opened or removed using microsurgical techniques similar to those used to reverse a vasectomy.

If nerve or spinal cord injury makes voluntary ejaculation impossible, a special technique using vibratory stimulation applied to the penis can produce a reflex ejaculation that can be used with assisted reproductive technologies to impregnate a woman.

Although not directly tied to infertility, some research has shown that extended bicycle riding using a bike seat that is not designed for the male anatomy can produce either temporary or long-lasting numbing of the penis and consequent erectile dysfunction. In some cases, damage to the arteries feeding the penis has also been observed after extended bike riding. Many types of bike seats are now available with a groove or indentation down the center to reduce the risk of such injury.

Congenital Abnormalities

Sometimes infertility is caused by problems that are present at birth (congenital). Here are some of the more common abnormalities:

- Congenital absence of the vas deferens is a rare condition in which testicular function is normal but the vas deferens are not present to conduct sperm to the ejaculate.

- About 1 in every 500 boys is born with the urethral opening not in its normal position at the tip of the penis, a condition called "hypospadias." Instead, the opening is on the lower side of the penis and may be any distance away from the tip. In such cases semen is not deposited at the back of a woman's vagina during unprotected sex, and thus fertility is impaired.

- Kallmann syndrome is a failure of a brain structure called the hypothalamus to produce gonadotropin-releasing hormone (GnRH). Without GnRH a man's pituitary is never properly controlled, which leads to a failure of the pituitary to secrete the hormones necessary for the production of both sperm and testosterone.

- Klinefelter syndrome occurs when an extra X chromosome is present in a man's cells (men normally have a single X and a single Y chromosome in each body cell). Men with Klinefelter syndrome have a low testosterone level and usually produce no or very few sperm, though the other effects of the condition are often so subtle they go unnoticed. Such men typically have small, poorly functioning testicles but have normal orgasms and ejaculations.

These various conditions can all be overcome by surgery, hormone replacement therapy, or assisted reproductive technology with extraction of sperm from the testicles or epididymis.

Medications to Boost Sperm Production

If a man's sperm count is low (a condition technically called "oligozoospermia") because of hormonal irregularities, a medication such as clomiphene citrate or tamoxifen may help. As noted in Chapter 2, clomiphene citrate (marketed under the names Clomid and Serophene) and tamoxifen (sold as Nolvadex) belong to a class of medications known as anti-estrogens, or selective estrogen receptor modulators (SERMs). In Chapter 2, I discussed taking these drugs as a way to boost testosterone, but several studies have shown that they can also improve sperm count and/or sperm motility in men.

Recall that the drugs work by boosting the output of GnRH from the hypothalamus. This, in turn, stimulates the pituitary gland to release more follicle-stimulating hormone (which encourages sperm production) and luteinizing hormone (which raises testosterone levels). Both of these functions are important because testosterone works indirectly to boost sperm count. The added sex drive produced by the testosterone may also increase a man's interest in sex, which may indirectly help his chances of conceiving.

As noted earlier, the main advantage of both clomiphene citrate and tamoxifen is that they work *with* the body's hormonal systems rather than clobbering those systems with external doses of pure testosterone. As noted earlier, even though testosterone replacement therapy can be valuable for men with an abnormally low testosterone level, it can actually impair their fertility because their bodies respond to the extra testosterone by shutting down the entire hormonal sequence, which impairs both natural testosterone production and sperm manufacture.

Nonetheless, for men with a low sperm count, these medications have been shown in preliminary studies to improve sperm count and function. Whether this translates into an actual increase in pregnancy rates hasn't been determined, but it makes sense that it would.[7] Since long-term studies of these medications have not been conducted in men, it is prudent for men to watch for signs of prostate cancer by having regular blood tests for prostate-specific antigen (PSA), which can suggest the presence of cancer.

Intrauterine Insemination (IUI)

Intrauterine insemination is the deposition of semen directly into a woman's uterus, using a thin tube. IUI can increase the chances of fertilization, particularly if a man has a low semen volume. Remember that seminal fluid transports sperm to the uterus. If the volume is low, using IUI can overcome the lack of fluid. IUI is also appropriate when the man's semen is normal but the doctor suspects that there may be a problem with his partner's cervix (the "gate" between the back of the vagina and the uterus). Sometimes, for example, a woman's cervical mucus does not thin as it should around the time she ovulates, which prevents sperm deposited in the vagina from swimming up into her uterus.

To increase the chance of conception, IUI is sometimes used in conjunction with ovulation-stimulating drugs. The insemination procedure, which is usually only mildly uncomfortable for the woman, is performed in a doctor's office at the time of ovulation or after the "trigger" injection of ovulation-stimulating medication is given. The man produces a semen sample by masturbation either at home or at the clinic, and the sperm are separated (or "washed") to select out the most energetically mobile sperm. Sperm washing also cleanses the sperm of potentially toxic chemicals that may cause adverse reactions in the uterus. A soft tube called a catheter is passed through the vagina and cervix, and the concentrated semen is deposited into the uterus.

Techniques for Special Cases

Many surgical and nonsurgical treatments exist for relatively uncommon causes of infertility, such as damage to the reproductive tract from accidents, inability to ejaculate because of nerve damage, or congenital anatomical defects. Sometimes these techniques are used in tandem with assisted reproductive technologies, for example, when electrical stimulation is used to create an artificial ejaculation and the semen thus obtained is used for *in vitro* fertilization. Although space does not permit an exhaustive description of these many techniques, men with less common causes of infertility should seek an expert in male fertility, because even in extreme cases, technology has improved to the point that real hope exists for fathering a child.

5

Finding Sperm When a Man Is "Sterile"

Katie is a physician's assistant at a big-city fertility clinic. Seeing so many couples with fertility problems every day made her a bit paranoid about getting pregnant herself, and so before she and her husband, Alex, began trying for a child they decided to undergo some preliminary tests just to be sure everything was fine.

Alex vividly remembers when Katie called from work with the results.

"You won't believe this, but they looked at the sample you gave them this morning and there's nothing there," she said. "No sperm, not one."

"I said, 'What?' And she said, 'We'll run the test again, but there's nothing there.' It was completely shocking and very depressing."

A second test confirmed the dismal result. Alex was one of

the roughly 20 percent of infertile men with so-called unexplained testicular failure. What we didn't yet know was whether there were some sperm in Alex's abnormally small testicles that were simply not making it out and up the vas deferens as they should. The only way to tell for sure is a surgical biopsy. If sperm are found in a biopsy, of course, it is best to retrieve them and use them immediately, so I advised Alex and Katie to prepare for *in vitro* fertilization (IVF). When Katie ovulated and was ready for the procedure, we would do the biopsy. If we found sperm, we would use them, but if we didn't, we would use sperm from a donor. To increase the chances for success, I put Alex on clomiphene citrate, which stimulated his sperm production.

"The hardest part for me," Alex says, "was knowing that the doctor was going to look for sperm from me but meanwhile my wife is preparing herself and having eggs retrieved and if they don't find sperm they'll have to go with donor sperm immediately. And that was a horrible thought for me. It brought up all kinds of issues—masculine things that pop into my head, like feeling I'm inadequate or something. It's really stressful."

The stress that Alex and Katie were feeling is extremely common. Fertility problems strike very deep emotional chords in both men and women and can generate intense, unpredictable, and surprising emotions. Like many couples, Alex and Katie found going to some sessions with a trained therapist to be extremely helpful.

"We found a psychologist who specializes in fertility issues," Alex says. "We met with her about once a week and discussed the emotions we had, what we were thinking, and anticipating what we'd do if we had to go with donor sperm. Would we tell our friends? Tell the kids? Would we keep it all a secret? It was useful for me to bounce these things off of someone other than my wife."

On a gray Saturday morning in March, Alex and Katie drove to the hospital for the biopsy and sperm extraction procedure. After he was prepped and unconscious, I removed a sample of Alex's testicular tissue and looked at it under a microscope: sperm! I harvested as much as I could, then gave the tiny vial to Katie's fertility clinic, where the sperm were put into special nutrients to boost their health and help them mature. The next day, twelve mature eggs were retrieved from Katie and each was injected with Alex's sperm. Six of the twelve were fertilized and began growing.

"We took the aggressive route and put all six back in," Alex says.

Now they could only wait to see if any of the six implanted themselves in Katie's uterus and began to grow. Several weeks later, her pregnancy test was positive. A little while later, an ultrasound found one embryo. Later ultrasounds found four, and the doctors recommended a selective reduction, meaning the removal of some embryos to allow the others a better chance of survival and reduce the risks to Katie that would be involved with carrying multiple fetuses to term, such as high blood pressure and gestational diabetes.

Before they made that decision, however, Katie started to

bleed heavily while driving to work one day. She feared she had lost them all, but ultrasound showed that two remained. Nature had done the reduction for her.

Katie carried the twins for thirty-one weeks, the last eight spent on bed rest. When she began to have contractions she entered the hospital, and for three days medications staved off the rhythmic pulses. But finally the drugs could not hold the contractions at bay, and she delivered via cesarean section. Both babies—a boy and a girl—came out breathing on their own with no major problems. Both are now happy, healthy infants.

"This whole thing turned from a terrible experience to one of the best in our lives," Alex says. "Our relationship as a couple has aged ten years, and we've only been married three years. But I appreciate the kids more than if it had been an easy road. When you have to fight for your kids this much and go through hell to get them, it feels very rewarding."

Using *in Vitro* Fertilization

Since 1981, when it was introduced in the United States, IVF and associated reproductive technologies have given hope to tens of thousands of couples who previously would not have been able to have genetically related children. The use of IVF has been steadily rising over the years. In 2001, for example (the last year for which data were available at this writing), about 107,000 cycles of IVF were conducted, which led to 29,344 live births and almost 41,000 babies.[1] In 2001, there

were 421 IVF clinics in the United States, most of them concentrated on the East and West Coasts (some western states
don't have a single clinic within their borders), and the industry is expanding rapidly.

It's important to point out that IVF is not the wonder technology it is sometimes made out to be. The fact is that more couples do *not* end up with a baby after IVF than do. The chance of
having a baby after a single IVF cycle in 2001 was 27 percent,
which is actually higher than the "success" rate of having a baby
via intercourse in any given menstrual period (a healthy couple
has about a 21 percent chance of conceiving in a given cycle). But
the chance of having a baby after two IVF cycles is only 47 percent—and since most couples stop the process after two cycles,
this means that most couples don't end up with a child. Couples
stop the process for many reasons, but most commonly because
it's expensive (roughly $12,000 per cycle), emotionally draining,
and logistically cumbersome.[2] If a couple is persistent and has the
financial resources to continue IVF after two cycles, their overall chances of having a baby improve to 61 percent after three
cycles and 72 percent after four cycles.

In addition, using IVF greatly increases the chances that a
woman will have twins or triplets. The rate of multiple live
births among women using IVF is about 37 percent, compared to only 3 percent in the general U.S. population.

These averages, however, mask some important details
related to the male and female biological clocks. If the success
rate is broken down by the age of the woman, a clear trend

becomes apparent: the chance of a successful pregnancy and delivery drops rapidly as the age of the woman rises above thirty-two.

It's very likely, given all we know, that paternal age also plays a strong role in the declining IVF pregnancy rates with age, but the studies we need to confirm this have not yet been completed.

Alex and Katie's story illustrates some themes common to most couples going through IVF—for example, their roller-coaster emotions and heightened anxiety at each hurdle in the process. Their story also highlights the fact that IVF is relatively demanding of the woman and not always comfortable. Hormones to prepare a woman's eggs must be given on a strict schedule, often by injection at home. And because women

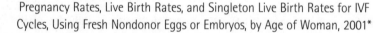

Pregnancy Rates, Live Birth Rates, and Singleton Live Birth Rates for IVF Cycles, Using Fresh Nondonor Eggs or Embryos, by Age of Woman, 2001*

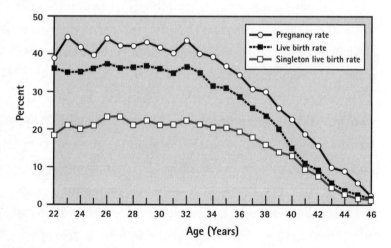

*For consistency, all rates are based on cycles started.

undergoing IVF are considered to be at high risk for complications, they must undergo more frequent diagnostic tests than normal.

But Alex and Katie's story also shows that hope exists even where there is an extreme condition, such as the complete lack of sperm in a man's semen. This impressive technology is constantly being improved, and today it is more widely available, more often covered by insurance, and more successful than ever, although, as just noted, it is still very expensive.

Making the decision to pursue IVF can be easy or difficult, depending on your circumstances. It's always important to explore all other avenues first, including getting thorough examinations of both partners by qualified doctors and following up with any of the "low-tech" treatment options discussed in the previous chapter. If these have failed, or if, as in Alex and Katie's case, a diagnosis is so clear that no other techniques could work, then it's time to take the plunge into IVF—if the couple can afford it.

Although IVF is an important option for the treatment of infertility, the decision to use IVF involves many factors in addition to success rates and cost. Going through repeated IVF cycles requires a substantial commitment of time, effort, money, and emotional energy. Therefore, a couple should carefully examine all related financial, psychological, and medical issues before beginning treatment. A couple should also consider the location of the clinic, the counseling and support services available, and the rapport that staff members have with their patients.

IVF is a large subject. Because this book is focused on the male biological clock, I will not go into elaborate detail about the many aspects of IVF related to the female side of the equation. Excellent information is available on this topic from both the American Urological Association and the American Society for Reproductive Medicine (see the appendix for contact information and Web sites). Here I will discuss IVF in broad strokes in order to give couples who may be grappling with male infertility enough information to guide further discussions with their physicians.

In Vitro Fertilization

Two basic IVF techniques account for 98 percent of all procedures done today: IVF and IVF with intracytoplasmic sperm injection (ICSI). Two much less common "cousins" of IVF, gamete intrafallopian transfer (GIFT) and zygote intrafallopian transfer (ZIFT), are covered at the end of this chapter.

In vitro fertilization involves harvesting ripe eggs from the woman and combining them with a man's sperm outside the body. IVF requires careful planning and timing to ensure that the woman's body is at maximum readiness for the procedure. IVF is appropriate for a wide range of problems, including blocked fallopian tubes, severe male infertility, or when no problem can be found but a couple is still infertile (called "idiopathic infertility").

An IVF cycle typically begins when a woman takes ovulation-stimulating drugs to prepare her uterus and increase the number of mature eggs that can be retrieved, though the procedure can also be done with eggs donated by another woman. Sometimes a healthy woman may choose to avoid ovarian stimulation, in which case her natural menstrual cycle is carefully monitored for signs of ovulation.

When it's likely that eggs are available, one or more are retrieved through a small puncture in the vagina. The eggs are then combined with sperm in the laboratory. If fertilization is successful, one or more of the resulting embryos are selected for transfer to the uterus. If one or more of the transferred embryos implant within the woman's uterus, the cycle then progresses to clinical pregnancy. If all goes well, the pregnancy progresses to the delivery of one or more infants. A cycle may be discontinued at any step for specific medical reasons (e.g., no eggs are produced or the embryo transfer was not successful) or by the patient's choice.

Intracytoplasmic Sperm Injection (ICSI)

In normal fertilization, thousands or millions of sperm swarm around an egg, but usually only one successfully penetrates the egg's outer shell to achieve a conception. With ICSI, a *single* sperm is selected, prepared, and then microsurgically injected into an egg. This is a technically demanding but valuable process for men with an extremely low sperm count or even, as in Alex's case, no sperm in the ejaculate at all. ICSI is used in almost half of all IVF procedures, and the rate of live births among couples who use ICSI due to male infertility is just slightly lower than the success rate of couples who use IVF without ICSI. In other words, the technique works well, and it successfully overcomes problems associated with severe male-factor infertility.

Sperm for ICSI are obtained either from normal ejaculation (via masturbation) or from sperm extraction directly from the epididymis or testicle using one of the biopsy techniques reviewed in Chapter 4. Sperm extraction is performed under local or general anesthesia and is usually only moderately uncomfortable. Using either a scalpel or a spring-loaded device that retrieves a core of tissue, the surgeon removes testicular tissue and examines it under a microscope for sperm. If suitable sperm are found, enough tissue is removed to ensure an adequate number for ICSI and the incisions are closed. If the sperm are not going to be used immediately, they are frozen for later use (see page 139 for details about sperm preservation).

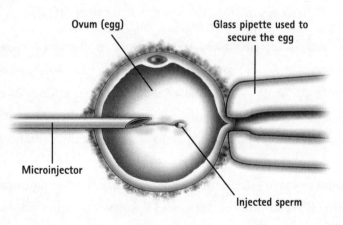

ICSI Technique

The semen or sperm is then prepared to select the most mobile sperm possible and to keep them healthy in a nourishing chemical environment. One (or typically more) eggs are retrieved from a woman's ovary following the procedures described earlier in this chapter. Each egg is then located under a microscope and held firmly while an extremely fine hollow glass needle is used to puncture the egg and inject the sperm. The entire process is conducted under high-power magnification and with special instruments to allow micromanipulation of both egg and sperm.

After sperm injection, the eggs are incubated for sixteen to eighteen hours, then examined for evidence of fertilization or signs of damage. Undamaged, fertilized embryos can then either be transferred back to the woman's uterus using standard IVF techniques or frozen for transfer at a later time.

If more than one egg is put into the uterus, the possibility of a viable pregnancy increases, but so does the chance of having twins, triplets, or even more babies. Multiple fetuses, however, are at significantly higher risk for a host of potential problems and increase the risk that the mother will experience complications as well. Because of this, if more than two eggs successfully implant and begin to grow, physicians usually recommend a selective reduction to allow the remaining two embryos a better chance of being carried to term while reducing the risk to the mother. Selective reduction is typically performed by injecting an embryo with a drug that stops further development. The procedure carries a small risk for miscarriage, but the risk is small compared to the risk posed by multiple fetuses. Women often feel conflicted, anxious, or guilty about the selective reduction process, but one study showed that several weeks afterward, 93 percent of women felt they would make the same decision again.[3]

Once the embryo or embryos are implanted and begin to grow, pregnancy proceeds normally, though usually women using IVF undergo more frequent monitoring because they are considered to be at higher risk for miscarriage.

GIFT and ZIFT

Two variations on IVF are occasionally used to overcome specific abnormalities in a woman's reproductive tract. Gamete intrafallopian transfer involves using a fiber-optic instrument called a laparoscope to guide the transfer of unfertilized eggs and sperm (gametes) into the woman's fallopian tubes through small incisions in her abdomen. Zygote intrafallopian transfer involves fertilizing a woman's eggs in the laboratory and then using a laparoscope to guide the transfer of the fertilized eggs (zygotes) into her fallopian tubes. GIFT or ZIFT are necessary only very rarely. Only about 1 percent of couples undergoing IVF uses either of these techniques.

"Adopting" Sperm

If a man has come to terms with the fact that he has no viable sperm in either his ejaculate or his testes, the couple may consider insemination with "adopted" sperm—that is, sperm donated by another man. A little-known fact is that more babies are born in this country using adopted donor sperm than from IVF. I use the term "adopted sperm" to better define what's really happening and to ease the emotional stress associated with the term "donor sperm." Couples can adopt sperm just as they can adopt children, but it is easier and usually less expensive. In this way the mother has a chance to have a child who is biologically related to her and gets to experience pregnancy, birth, nursing, and all the other aspects of motherhood. The male partner has the chance to participate in this process as well. The nine-month process of pregnancy and then labor and delivery is a significantly different experience from adopting a baby, which is why some couples choose this method.

Couples can usually "adopt" sperm based on donor criteria such as ethnic group, educational level or profession, hair color, eye color, sperm count or motility, and other pertinent information. Couples usually select a donor who resembles the male partner. Both donors and their sperm are tested for diseases such as HIV and hepatitis. If a woman has normal reproductive functioning, the thawed and prepared donor sperm is put into her uterus using intrauterine insemination techniques at the time of her ovulation. If the woman's reproductive functioning is compromised in some way, donor sperm can be used with IVF or ICSI as well. The pregnancy success rate with adopted (donor) sperm and intrauterine insemination (the most common arrangement) is approximately 10 to 15 percent for each insemination, which is lower than the rate in any given month of healthy men and women trying to conceive via intercourse. The reason is that the sperm is frozen and then thawed, and frozen sperm are less viable than fresh.

In his story earlier in this chapter, Alex gives voice to the common initial reluctance on the part of men to the idea of using donor sperm. It's a natural reluctance, but that doesn't mean it's entirely rational or even in a man's long-term self-interest. Another patient of mine, a man with testicular failure who turned to donor sperm to have two children with his wife, puts it this way.

"It was a little difficult at first," he says. "But it's a question of whether you want children or not. We had a choice of adopting a baby or adopting sperm and having my wife proceed with pregnancy. I knew my wife wanted to experience pregnancy, and she was more enthusiastic about adopting sperm than adopting a baby. Once I had understood that I had no sperm and no chance of conceiving a baby, the decision was easier. And it doesn't make any difference to me now that my kids are not genetically related to me. I am their father, and they are my children. I love my children beyond love, and I wouldn't change anything about what I did."

It's my experience that men decide to adopt sperm once they have exhausted all options and have found a degree of closure about the situation.

Preserving Sperm

Some men have advance warning of infertility: those diagnosed with cancer, particularly testicular cancer, the treatment of which is known to damage or destroy fertility. These men should bank their own sperm before they begin their cancer treatment. The rapid advances in IVF mean they have a good chance of having genetically related children once their cancer is in remission.

When sperm are stored properly and frozen at extremely low temperatures (cryopreservation) viability can be maintained for years or decades. Pregnancies have been reported using sperm that was stored for twenty years prior to thawing and insemination.

A Message to Men

It can be all too easy during IVF procedures for men to feel like bit players in the larger drama. Even though men can be intimately involved—as was Alex, who took medications prior to sperm extraction and then underwent a surgical procedure to obtain the sperm—the focus of both doctors and fertility clinics tends to be on the woman. This attention is understandable, of course: it's the woman who must bear the burden of pregnancy, diagnostic tests, and any interventions required to keep the fetus (or fetuses) from being born prematurely. And it's simply true that, in some respects, men are *always* spectators to pregnancy, labor, and delivery, whether they use IVF or not.

But men do play—or, at least, *should* play—a vital role in the process. Particularly when a woman is going through an IVF cycle, men can provide essential emotional and logistical support. To the extent that a man involves himself in the nitty-gritty details of such things as mixing hormone preparations for home injection or accompanying the woman to checkups or tests, he will become a true partner in the entire procedure. For most men, logistical support is relatively easy, emotional support often more difficult. Being true to your own needs and feelings while simultaneously trying to support, listen to, and really appreciate your partner can be a very delicate balancing act, particularly if, as often happens, things don't go completely smoothly. Setbacks, such as failed cycles or miscarriage, are relatively common, and the moods of both partners at such time can swing precipitously. Couples who are unprepared for such swings and the emotional stress that can accompany infertility in general—and IVF in particular—can be in for a rough ride.

Chapter 7 delves into this issue in more detail, with an emphasis on the male perspective, and contains many practical suggestions for dealing effectively with the emotional side of both infertility and sexual performance problems such as erectile dysfunction.

6

Slowing the Biological Clock: A Guide to Sexual Health

A man's genes, coupled with his life circumstances, set the broad limits of his sexual biological clock. In other words, the quality of his semen and his sperm, his average testosterone level, and the quality of his erections are controlled, to a large extent, by his unique genetic heritage. But men can still do a lot to improve their fertility and their sexual performance. In this chapter, I'll look at general ways that any man can slow or reverse his biological clock and improve his sexual health. Following these guidelines will absolutely make a difference, regardless of your age or whether you have any current problems. Remember that sexual anatomy is a lot like a fairly complicated machine, and, like any machine, it will perform better if it is used properly and maintained regularly. Both men and their partners should consider what follows an instruction manual for the care and upkeep of the male sexual anatomy.

Eat the Proper Fuel,
Do the Proper Amount of Exercise

The old cliché "You are what you eat" contains a fair amount of truth. A man's body, including his sex organs, is made from the food he eats, the beverages he drinks, and the air he breathes. Eat right, and everything improves—including sexual health. As with most things in life, an appropriate guide for eating to promote sexual health is "All things in moderation, including excess." The idea is to avoid extremes in any direction and yet preserve the pleasure of eating.

For example, much research shows that a high-fat diet, high cholesterol levels, and obesity lower testosterone levels and increase the risk of erection problems. That's because excess fat is converted to estrogenlike compounds that curtail the production of testosterone, and fat in the blood can clog the small arteries that feed the penis. Remember, what is bad for the heart is bad for the penis. A recent study, in fact, found that, conversely, improving cardiac health improves erections, a fact recently illustrated by a study showing improved erectile function in a group of men treated with a cholesterol-lowering medication.[1]

On the other hand, studies also show that very lean men—for example, marathon runners—have lower-than-average testosterone levels. That's because the compound used to build testosterone molecules in the body is cholesterol, and extreme exercise lowers cholesterol levels to abnormal levels. A man needs enough cholesterol in his diet to maintain testosterone production, but not so much that it produces body fat or clogged arteries.

A similar dynamic exists with vitamins and minerals. Many studies in both animals and men show that deficiencies of vitamin E, vitamin B_{12}, zinc, selenium, and a host of other vitamins reduce sperm production. But that doesn't mean guys should go out and start popping extra zinc tablets. Taking megadoses of any vitamin can cause problems—the body is simply not built to absorb such large amounts, and a man will both be wasting money and harming his health by doing so. Men need *adequate* levels of all the key vitamins, particularly the so-called antioxidant vitamins A, C, and E. Although the current recommended levels of these and other vitamins and minerals may not be perfect (they are revised periodically in light of new research), I think it makes sense to follow the latest recommendations and take a general-purpose vitamin supplement every day that will "cover your bases."

Here are the latest dietary guidelines for men published by the National Research Council. This is the best guide for determining if you are eating enough of a given nutrient, such as fiber, and for determining how much, if any, vitamin and mineral supplements you need.

Total daily calories	2,300
Total fat	76 grams (g)
Cholesterol	No more than 300 milligrams (mg)
Sodium (salt)	No more than 2,400 mg
Dietary fiber	20–30 g
Protein	63 g
Vitamin A	900 micrograms (µg)
Vitamin C	90 mg
Vitamin D	10 µg (equivalent to 400 international units [IU])
Vitamin E	15 mg
Calcium	1,200 mg
Iron	10 mg
Zinc	15 mg
Beta-carotene	5–6 mg
Folate	400 µg

Of course, it would be best if we all derived an optimal vitamin and mineral balance every day from the foods we eat, but that's not always easy or possible these days. A supplement is particularly important for vegetarians or those on other limited diets because, unless one is very careful, vitamin and mineral deficiencies can occur.

Science has not found any particular diet that reliably

improves testosterone or fertility. Everything points to the general idea that if a man eats for whole-body health, he'll be eating for his sexual health as well. The following guidelines are recommended.

- "No wheat, no weight." Limit wheat products such as breads, pizza, pasta, cookies, and cake.

- Avoid white flours, white rice, and sugar; all these cause large spikes in blood sugar levels that can sap energy and lead to adult-onset diabetes. Whole grains are far preferable (and are often more tasty as well).

- Switch from saturated fats such as butter to unsaturated fats such as liquid oils.

- Eat plenty of fruits and vegetables (just don't drown them in butter or salad dressing).

- Keep portions of protein, particularly red meat, modest.

- Get more fiber in your diet. A morning high-fiber cereal is a very good way to help reach the recommended level.

- Eat a diet that is balanced in protein, carbohydrates, and fats; you'll feel less hungry. In general, consumption of carbohydrates increases appetite, while consumption of fats and proteins decreases appetite—but don't push this to extremes.

These guidelines may sound overly simple, but you don't need to follow complicated regimens, fancy diets, or other faddish ideas such as a low-carb diet, a low-protein diet, or a low-fat diet. Most people instinctively know how to eat well; the problem is not succumbing to the temptations produced by our inborn cravings for fat and sweets, cravings that served our species very well ten thousand years ago but are now causing us grief.

Optimal sexual health is also promoted by moderate, regular exercise. Again, the key is avoiding extremes. Studies show that men who exercise strenuously (i.e., men who run more than 100 miles a week or who bicycle more than 50 miles a week) usually have a lower testosterone level than men who exercise more moderately. Given that most men do not, in fact, exercise even moderately, this is not exactly a huge public health problem. Exercise at any level, even walking, is better than no exercise, but maximum benefit is derived when exercise is strenuous enough to be aerobic, meaning any activity that uses large muscle groups, can be maintained continuously, and is rhythmic in nature. Such activity causes the heart and lungs to work harder than normal, which is the key to achieving both the physical and mental advantages of exercise.

When an overweight man, particularly one with excess abdominal fat, has a low testosterone level (which often is the case), I do not recommend that he begin exercising right away. It's simply going to be frustrating because he will lack the drive and energy needed to exercise. Instead, I boost his testosterone levels medically, and almost always, he then finds he *wants* to exercise because it simply feels good. Exercise may cause an initial small weight gain from added muscle mass, but this is usually followed (in overweight men) by significant weight loss, because more calories will be burned and the added muscle mass raises a man's metabolic rate.

Men need to think about their sexual health when they're making choices about which foods to eat and whether or not to exercise. It's one thing for a man to know in the abstract that it's good to exercise and eat right; it's quite another to understand that doing so will help his sex life and potency.

Quit Smoking

Several studies show that men who smoke have lower sperm counts and their sperm are somewhat more likely to be abnormally shaped. Smoking also makes it harder to get and maintain an erection because it releases (among other things) adrenaline and other stimulating compounds that make it harder for blood to flow into the penis in response to sexual stimulation. Smoking is one of the major risk factors for erectile dysfunction.

Clearly, however, smoking by itself doesn't cause infertility, nor does it make sex impossible—if it did, the tobacco industry would be out of business very quickly! Smoking is just one of many lifestyle habits that when added together can significantly erode fertility or sexuality.

Avoid Anabolic Steroids

As we saw in Chapter 2, more and more men these days are using anabolic steroids to gain a competitive edge or become "bulked up." Anabolic steroids act like testosterone in the body. Taking the doses commonly used by athletes is like flooding the body with extra testosterone, which cripples a man's natural testosterone production and fertility. Although some athletes take steroids in six- to twelve-week cycles, resting in between in order to "give their bodies time to recover," it actually takes between six months and a year for sperm and testosterone production to return to normal after a course of steroid use. Anabolic steroids are simply bad for fertility—and ultimately bad for your overall health. (Note that corticosteroid medications such as prednisone and cortisone, which are used to relieve itching, rashes, allergic reactions, and other medical conditions, are *not* the same as anabolic steroids and have no effect on either fertility or sexuality.)

Avoid Hot Tubs

Hot tubs are great, and if all a man cares about is sex, there's no harm done and possibly plenty of good to come from a nice relaxing soak (particularly if it's done with a partner). Unfortunately, as mentioned earlier, heat and sperm are a bad mix. Sperm are made in the testicles, which usually hang from the body in the scrotum. As we've seen, the sperm-making cells of the testicles don't work right unless they are *cooler* than body temperature by a few degrees Fahrenheit. In order to keep the temperature of the testicles relatively constant, the scrotum is lined with temperature-sensitive muscles. In warm conditions the muscles relax and let the testicles hang far from the body, whereas cold temperatures (particularly cold water) make the scrotum contract, pulling the testicles tight against the body for added warmth. Soaking in a hot tub makes it impossible for the testicles to remain as cool as they would like to be, which may reduce sperm formation or harm sperm that are already made. (This impact on fertility also occurs if a man is running a high fever.)

Avoid Drugs

Abuse or long-term heavy use of alcohol, marijuana, cocaine, or practically any other recreational drug clearly impairs both fertility and sexual performance. As Shakespeare wryly noted in *Macbeth,* alcohol "provokes the desire, but it takes away the performance." The same can be said for other drugs when used to excess.

But the jury is still out about whether occasional or moderate use of drugs has any kind of significant long-term effects on reproductive health. Although animal studies and research with relatively high doses of THC (the active ingredient in marijuana) have shown a negative effect on such factors as sperm quality and quantity, a recent report by the Institute of Medicine says: "It remains to be determined whether smoked marijuana or oral THC taken in prescribed doses has a clinically significant effect on the fertilizing capacity of human sperm."[2] In addition to this, the report notes that studies of marijuana's effects on fertility "have yielded conflicting results." The situation with alcohol is similar: effects can be demonstrated at high doses or in alcoholics, but the evidence is mixed at the levels most people consume.

Common sense suggests that men with fertility or erectile problems should abstain from, or indulge only very moderately in, alcohol or other recreational drugs.

Check Your Medications

Many medications commonly used to treat other illnesses or conditions can affect fertility or sexuality. As noted in previous chapters, some antidepressants impair erection and make it difficult or impossible to achieve an orgasm. (Of course, as we saw in Chapter 3, this can be an advantage for men with premature ejaculation.) Other medications degrade sperm quality. Here's a list of the major classes of drugs that have the potential to harm sexual health:

- Calcium channel blockers, beta-blockers, and thiazide medications for high blood pressure
- Cimetidine (for peptic ulcers)
- Cyclosporin (after an organ transplant)

- Chemotherapy for cancer
- Antidepressants of the selective serotonin reuptake inhibitor (SSRI) class

Men who suspect that they are experiencing an adverse sexual reaction to a drug should talk to their doctor as soon as possible about switching to another drug or changing their dose.

The preceding advice in this chapter can help *every* man, whether he's experiencing a problem or not. Remember: what's good for your heart is good for your sexual health, and anything that improves your overall health will improve both your fertility and your sexual performance.

7

Working as a Team

About two weeks after his divorce papers were made final, Erik accepted an invitation from friends to a dinner party. There he met Kris, also divorced, and they fell in love.

"After about four or five months I knew in my head and my heart that she was the person for me," Erik says.

There was just one problem: Kris had no children and now wanted them badly. Erik was all for it, even though he had two grown children of his own. But after the birth of his second child, he had a vasectomy.

"My ex-wife and I were content with two kids and thought we were content with each other," Erik says. "I figured we were done—I was married, I had two kids, a house, you know, the classic American story."

So Erik went back to the doctor who had performed his vasectomy to have it reversed. The doctor had not performed very many of these procedures.

"I think we went into it thinking, 'Hey, you just go in there and have everything undone, what's the big deal?'" he says. "We simplified what I now know is a very complicated scenario."

The surgery cost Erik about $7,500 and lasted almost five hours. But three months later the first semen analysis found no viable sperm. Another three months passed, and again, no sperm. The reversal had failed.

"I think it hurt Kris more than me," he says. "I was disappointed, but she was *really* disappointed."

Despite that disappointment, Erik and Kris were married several months later.

"It was a confident move on her part," Erik says. "My wife is very determined. She simply would not accept failure in this arena. And also, I think, we both viewed our relationship as a couple as our primary focus—if we eventually had a child, fine, but we had a solid foundation with or without a child."

That foundation was tested by the *in vitro* fertilization (IVF) process, which they decided to pursue using sperm extraction from Erik's testicles and intracytoplasmic sperm injection (ICSI).

"It's a very exacting process," Erik says. "There's a lot of rushing around, a lot of mixing of different chemicals. We had to take classes, had to learn how to give injections in different parts of the body depending on what part of the cycle Kris was in. It's a lot of keeping track, getting prescriptions, watching videos. It was all-consuming."

Fortunately, Kris was healthy and seemed not to have any

problems. But she and Erik wouldn't know until the day of the sperm extraction procedure if Erik still had viable sperm in his testicles or epididymis.

"The first time I went in for an extraction was the most scary time," Erik says. "But Dr. Fisch took the sample, rushed into the back room to look at it, and when he came out he was practically cheering—he'd found plenty of sperm."

But their high hopes following the implantation came crashing down after it became clear that Kris wasn't pregnant.

"When you fail, it's very disheartening," Erik says. "Much more so than when the reversal failed because you have to put so much more time and energy into IVF."

Undaunted, they waited and then began a second cycle. This time two embryos took and were robust enough that, at Thanksgiving, Erik and Kris told close family members she was pregnant with twins. Then, on an exam in the weeks before Christmas, the doctor saw that the embryos had stopped maturing and would have to be removed.

"That was the hardest time of all," Erik says. "That was bottom. I was surprised that I cried in the doctor's office. My wife was also very upset. It was the lowest point that we collectively went through together in the process, and it really showed me that this wasn't just a medical experience we were going through, it was a psychological experience. And if I have a criticism of IVF centers, it's that they don't put as much energy into psychological support as they do on the medical side of it."

Despite the mounting costs, the gnawing doubts, the discomfort of the sperm extraction procedure, and the pain of disappointment, they went for another cycle.

This time a single embryo took, and it continued to grow as the months slowly passed. Each ultrasound, each checkup, each test for possible problems was stressful. In the end, it was a perfectly normal pregnancy. In labor, Kris dilated so rapidly the hospital personnel didn't have time to do an epidural, so she delivered without pain medications.

"When my son came out and he was healthy, I was immensely relieved," Erik says. "I felt the four years of waiting come off my shoulders. He was finally here! I was just so gratified."

It was after their son had begun toddling around on two feet that Kris tentatively told Erik she was thinking she would like to have another child.

"And I said, 'Oh, my God, I don't know if I can go through this again,'" he says. "But I didn't think about it too long before I said, 'Yes, if it means that much to you, okay.'"

They waited another year and then went back to the clinic and went through another cycle and another ride on the emotional roller coaster. But nothing took.

It was then that I brought up the possibility of correcting Erik's botched vasectomy reversal. The advantages, if it succeeded, were that it would allow them to "try" as many times as they'd like without the expense, inconvenience, and disruption of IVF cycles. They decided to give it a shot.

I performed a vasoepididymostomy, directly connecting the good end of Erik's vas deferens to his epididymis. I thought the operation went well, but only time would tell if it had worked.

Three months later Erik gave me a semen sample. His count was stellar, and the sperm looked great. Three months after that the numbers kept improving.

Erik and Kris are now, as of this writing, trying for their second child the old-fashioned way, which they're delighted about. But it can still be taxing, still be stressful, and still bring up powerful feelings.

"It's not as gut-wrenching as the IVF cycles," Erik says. "But it's still a challenge. The whole process has been one of the hardest things emotionally that I've ever experienced. It tests your relationship, tests your belief in God, tests a lot of things that most people don't give a second thought about."

Coping with Problems of
Male Infertility or Sexuality

Problems with male infertility or sexual performance are often extremely stressful for men and, if they have a partner, stressful on their relationship. Sex and sexuality are simply too strongly wired into human nature for it to be any other way. Even when a problem, from a medical standpoint, is relatively mild and easily fixed, such as minor erectile dysfunction that responds to an oral medication, from a psychological and emotional standpoint the problem can be fraught with difficulty. As we've seen, for example, erectile dysfunction typically sets in slowly and a couple may subtly change their sexual patterns, expectations, and feelings over the course of years. Fixing an erection in such cases is easy, but restoring a loving, mutually satisfying emotional climate surrounding sex takes time and energy.

When the problem is infertility, the stresses can be much more extreme, as Erik's story illustrates. The many complicated medical and financial decisions, the uncertainties surrounding any form of treatment, and the simple hassle of office visits, examinations, tests, and meetings can strain relationships to the breaking point. Add the extra sensitivity and emotional volatility produced by the hormones that a woman, man, or both may be taking as part of the treatment, and you have the potential for real emotional turmoil.

In general, I find that women are more skilled than men at coping with the emotional roller coaster of male sexual problems. That's hardly surprising, since men, by nature, tend to be less emotionally intelligent than women and approach problems from a more analytical, "how-can-I-fix-it?" point of view. Since much has been written about the female side of infertility and how women can cope with the emotions they face, I'm going to concentrate here on some advice for the men, gleaned during my years of helping men through the process.

Most couples who are dealing with any kind of male sexual

problem will benefit from at least a few sessions with a coun-selor or therapist. Your relationship doesn't need to be in cri-sis to see a therapist. Indeed, seeing a therapist when your relationship is *not* in crisis can help you both avoid serious problems. It's helpful to view therapy as a classroom—a place to learn more about your relationship, your partner, and your overall situation. It's a place to learn and practice valuable "peo-ple skills" that can really improve communication, intimacy, and satisfaction. Therapy can be especially helpful at certain key points in infertility treatment, such as deciding whether to pursue the option of adopting sperm or deciding whether or not to quit pursuing a treatment after repeated failures.

Therapists (and I use this term quite loosely to include psychiatrists, psychologists, counselors, social workers, and many other mental health professionals) usually specialize, and it is most helpful for issues of male sexuality to find a therapist with experience in sexuality, infertility, or the spe-cific kind of psychotherapy called interpersonal therapy, which deals specifically with relationship issues. Therapy need not be long-term; most of the time a great deal can be gained by six to twelve sessions of short-term, goal-oriented therapy. Your doctor may be able to suggest therapists in your area, or you can explore some of the organizations listed in the appendix, many of which offer services for locating thera-pists.

One of the simplest, yet most difficult, things a man can do to promote understanding, foster togetherness, and cope effectively with infertility is to listen to his partner. That probably sounds trivial, but it's not. It can be incredibly difficult, in the heat of an argument or emotionally loaded discussion, to avoid interrupting and to let your partner say what she wants to say no matter how "off base," "illogical," or "wrong" it may seem. Women don't necessarily want their partner to solve their "problem" or suggest ways to fix things—they just want him to listen to what they have to say and try to understand without passing judgment. Men should resist the temptation to interject, "correct," or debate. That doesn't mean not talking at all; it just means giving a woman the time to finish her thoughts completely before responding.

When dealing with sexuality or fertility problems, men tend to avoid talking about the issue with other men. So much of manhood revolves around sex and potency, and such strong biological drives are at work in the dynamic that even just admitting to another guy that you have a fertility problem can seem embarrassing or shameful even though, logically, it's no different from any other medical problem. But clamming up about the topic can be a real handicap. I always encourage men to talk to a brother, a father, a best friend, or a clergy member about what they're going though. It is comforting to be heard and helpful to air your true feelings away from your partner. It's also sometimes very helpful for a man to talk to another man who has already been through a particular procedure or process. (I should add that sometimes a man may simply not be ready to talk about it—and trying to force him to "open up" may be counterproductive. This pattern of male behavior can drive women crazy—understandably—but the solution is not to mount a frontal assault on his reticence. The partner of a man dealing with a sexual health issue should look for more subtle ways to encourage communication—and pick times when he is relaxed and undistracted.)

As stressful as the emotional roller coaster of infertility can be, it need not weaken a relationship or provoke psychological problems. In fact, couples who have worked through the ups and downs often say the experience has forced them to mature or grow in ways they might never have experienced otherwise. They embody the words of Nietzsche: "That which does not kill me makes me stronger."

Here are some suggestions to men for finding common ground with their partners, maintaining a sense of teamwork, and avoiding problems:

- Show support with actions in addition to words.
- Expect wide mood swings and unpredictable emotions.
- As often as possible, go to appointments together for "moral support," even if one partner is not technically involved.
- Consider attending meetings of infertility support groups.
- Don't threaten a partner with divorce if he or she refuses to pursue a particular option. If you feel "stuck" in a disagreement, back off, cool down, remind each other of the core values you both cherish, and then, if needed, take the

discussion to a therapist or counselor who has experience in dealing with infertility.

- Avoid placing blame; male sexual problems are nobody's fault, there are almost always physical problems at work, and nobody should feel guilty about them.

If Things Get Serious

The stresses and strains of male sexual problems can sometimes trigger full-blown anxiety, depression, or substance abuse. Sometimes the differences in beliefs, attitudes, or desires between partners are so stark and communication is so difficult that the relationship becomes truly endangered. In such a case, you both should seek help from a psychiatrist or psychologist. If medications are warranted for a problem, the psychiatrist, pharmacologist, or other doctor should be knowledgeable about male sexual problems, particularly male infertility, to avoid prescribing a treatment that would make the situation worse (such as giving a selective serotonin reuptake inhibitor [SSRI] antidepressant to a man experiencing erectile dysfunction).

Here are some signs and signals that should prompt a man to seek help for himself or his partner as quickly as possible:

- Loss of interest in usual activities
- Depressed mood that has lasted two weeks or longer
- Frequent fights that don't lead to resolution or agreement

- Difficulty thinking of anything other than infertility
- High anxiety levels
- Diminished ability to accomplish tasks
- Difficulty concentrating
- Altered sleep patterns (difficulty falling asleep or staying asleep, early-morning awakening, sleeping more than usual)
- Change (increase or decrease) in appetite or weight
- Increased use of drugs or alcohol
- Thoughts about death or suicide
- Social isolation
- Persistent feelings of pessimism, guilt, or worthlessness
- Persistent feelings of bitterness or anger

Sex

For most guys, the prospect of having sex without any birth control with the goal of conceiving a child sounds wonderful, particularly if it comes after many years of using birth control to *avoid* pregnancy. And it is wonderful—until the months drag on and what was once spontaneous, fun, and sexy ends up becoming . . . well, a chore. This can be true even for couples without a fertility issue, but it's particularly likely when a couple is in the midst of treatment. The pressure to "perform on cue" and to time intercourse to coincide with ovulation can also make it difficult for men to get and keep their erections (so-called performance anxiety), which can be very frustrating for both partners. The sheer work and stress involved in IVF or IVF with ICSI can also erode a couple's sex life.

It can take some attention and effort to restore a sex life during infertility treatment and afterward. The most important thing is to be able to talk about sex with your partner. It's very easy to have false assumptions about what your partner does or does not want. Maybe she doesn't want to have sex as much as you think she does—or maybe she's more frustrated than she lets on about the lack of sex. You have to talk to each other.

If you and your partner are having some difficulty or conflict with sex, it's often better to avoid tackling the problem head-on and instead concentrate on building up the feelings that may, in turn, lead to desire. First and foremost, that means a man should pay attention to his partner and demonstrate his love and affection. Little things count: back rubs, unexpected flowers, making a date (and arranging for a babysitter if needed), or just finding some time to talk about something more meaningful than the car, the bills, the dishes, and the state of the house. Of course, deliberate attempts to create a romantic mood won't hurt either—but such efforts must be subtle to work, otherwise they will feel forced or artificial. It's easy enough to light some candles, turn down the lights, or wear sexy underwear. It's usually a lot harder to muster the physical and emotional energy needed to make sex the relaxed, mutually enjoyable pleasure it was in the early days of the relationship.

If having sex begins to feel like a chore, it might help to consider the analogy of exercising. A lot of men and women have to make an effort to go to the gym, but once they get there and get into it, they enjoy it. Sex can be that way sometimes. You may not feel turned on or particularly sexy, but if you make an initial effort and begin, you may both find you get into it and enjoy it.

On a very practical note, when you are having sex to conceive a child, it's best to avoid any type of lubricant (even saliva), as these can block sperm from entering the cervix or make the chemical conditions of the vagina hazardous to the sperm's health. If vaginal dryness is an issue, try spending more time on foreplay or experiment with various types of erotica. Another option is to try natural lubricants such as canola oil or (believe it or not) egg whites.

I hope you find some of these suggestions helpful. The emotional and psychological dimensions of sexual problems are just as important as all of the medical and technical dimensions I've explored in the rest of the book. Rewinding the male biological clock is a real possibility for many men, and, as we've seen, problems with sexual performance or fertility can almost always be overcome. But everyone involved in the process must remember that men are more than erections or sperm-making machines and women are more than wombs. We are all deeply emotional beings (even if a lot of men don't show it), and we must pay attention to our emotional lives and care for ourselves and each other, particularly in times of difficulty or stress.

As we've seen throughout this book, many specific techniques are available to reverse a man's biological clock when his sexual or reproductive function is impaired. I hope the advice and information in this book will help both men and their partners better understand any problems with fertility or sexuality that they might be dealing with, and I hope the personal stories of some of my patients will give them hope. Remember: solutions exist for practically any sexual health problem. I wish couples the best in their efforts to achieve higher levels of sexual and reproductive health and sincerely hope this book has made those efforts a little easier.

APPENDIX

Finding Help

Dr. Harry Fisch
Male Reproductive Center of Columbia University/
New York Presbyterian Hospital
ADDRESS: 944 Park Avenue, New York, NY 10028
PHONE: (212) 879-0800
WEB ADDRESS: www.malebiologicalclock.com

American Association of Sex Educators, Counselors, and Therapists
ADDRESS: P.O. Box 5488, Richmond, VA 23220-0488
WEB ADDRESS: www.aasect.org

American Diabetes Association
ADDRESS: 1701 North Beauregard Street, Alexandria, VA 22311
PHONE: (800) DIABETES
WEB ADDRESS: www.diabetes.org

Sexual Function Health Council
American Foundation for Urologic Disease
ADDRESS: 1128 North Charles Street, Baltimore, MD 21201
PHONE: (800) 433-4215 or (410) 468-1800
E-MAIL: impotence@afud.org
WEB ADDRESS: www.impotence.org

The New York Center for Human Sexuality
Columbia University/ New York Presbyterian Hospital
Dr. Ridwan Shabsigh
ADDRESS: 161 Fort Washington Avenue, New York, NY 10032
PHONE: 212-305-0123
WEB ADDRESS: www.nychs.com

American Fertility Association
ADDRESS: 666 Fifth Avenue, Suite 278, New York, NY 10103
PHONE: (888) 917-3777
WEB ADDRESS: www.theafa.org

American Society for Reproductive Medicine
ADDRESS: 1209 Montgomery Highway, Birmingham, AL 35216-2809
PHONE: (205) 978-5000
WEB ADDRESS: www.asrm.org
(Includes a "find a doctor" service for locating fertility specialists
in your area.)

American Urological Association
ADDRESS: 1120 North Charles Street, Baltimore, MD 21201
PHONE: (410) 727-1100
E-MAIL: aua@auanet.org
WEB ADDRESS: www.auanet.org

RESOLVE: The National Infertility Association
ADDRESS: 1310 Broadway, Somerville, MA 02144
PHONE: (888) 623-0744
E-MAIL: info@resolve.org
WEB ADDRESS: www.resolve.org

Notes

Introduction: The Silent Epidemic

1. S. A. Kidd, B. Eskenazi, and A. J. Wyrobek, "Effects of Male Age on Semen Quality and Fertility: A Review of the Literature," *Fertility and Sterility* 75, no. 2 (2001): 237–248.
2. W. C. L. Ford, K. North, H. Taylor, et al., "Increasing Paternal Age Is Associated with Delayed Conception in a Large Population of Fertile Couples: Evidence for Declining Fecundity in Older Men," *Human Reproduction* 15, no. 8 (2000): 1703–1708.
3. R. H. Martin, A. W. Rademaker, K. Hildebrand, et al., "Variation in the Frequency and Type of Sperm Chromosomal Abnormalities Among Normal Men," *American Journal of Human Genetics* 77, no. 2 (October 1987): 108–114.
4. H. Fisch, G. Hyun, R. Golden, et al., "The Influence of Paternal Age on Down Syndrome," *Journal of Urology* 169, no. 6 (2003): 2275–2278.

1. The Male Biological Clock

1. B. Eskenazi, A. J. Wyrobek, E. Sloter, et al., "The Association of Age and Semen Quality in Healthy Men," *Human Reproduction* 18, no. 2 (February 2003): 447–454.

2. E. de la Rochebrochard and P. Thonneau, "Paternal Age and Maternal Age Are Risk Factors for Miscarriage: Results of a Multicentre European Study," *Human Reproduction* 17, no. 6 (2002): 1649–1656.

3. J. M. Dabbs, D. LaRue, and P. M. Williams, "Testosterone and Occupational Choice: Actors, Ministers, and Other Men," *Journal of Personality and Social Psychology* 59 (1990): 1261–1265.

4. H. A. Feldman, I. Goldstein, D. G. Hatzichristou, R. J. Krane, and J. B. McKinlay, "Impotence and Its Medical and Psychosocial Correlates: Results of the Massachusetts Male Aging Study," *The Journal of Urology* 151 (1994): 54–61.

5. From H. W. G. Baker, "Male Infertility," in *Endocrinology*, 4th ed., L. J. DeGroot and J. L. Jameson, chief editors (Philadelphia: W. B. Saunders Company, 2001), pp. 308–328.

2. The Truth About Testosterone

1. E. L. Rhoden and A. Morgentaler, "Risks of Testosterone-Replacement Therapy and Recommendations for Monitoring," *The New England Journal of Medicine* 350 (2004): 482–492.

2. S. Bhasin and J. G. Buckwalter, "Testosterone Supplementation in Older Men: A Rational Idea Whose Time Has Not Yet Come," *Journal of Andrology* 22 (2001): 718–731.

3. E. C. Tsai, A. M. Matsumoto, W. Y. Fujimoto, and E. J. Boyko, "Association of Bioavailable, Free, and Total Testosterone with Insulin Resistance," *Diabetes Care* 27 (2004): 861–868.

4. E. L. Rhoden and A. Morgentaler, "Risks of Testosterone-Replacement Therapy and Recommendations for Monitoring," *The New England Journal of Medicine* 350 (2004): 482–492.

5. A. T. Guay, S. Bansal, and G. J. Heatley, "Effect of Raising Endogenous Testosterone Levels in Impotent Men with Secondary Hypogonadism: Double Blind Placebo-Controlled Trial with Clomiphene Citrate," *Journal of Clinical Endocrinology and Metabolism* 80, no. 12 (1995): 3,546–3,552.

6. S. J. Segal and L. Mastroianni, *Hormone Use in Menopause and Male Andropause* (New York: Oxford University Press, 2003), pp. 116–118.

3. Viagra Generation

1. D. Sharlip, "New Therapies for Erectile Dysfunction. Medscape Urology," at www.medscape.com/viewarticle/459656, accessed February 2, 2004.

2. E. O. Laumann, A. Paik, and R. C. Rosen, "Sexual Dysfunction in the United States: Prevalence and Predictors," *The Journal of the American Medical Association* 281, no. 6 (1999): 537–544.

3. M. Atmaca, M. Kuloglu, E. Tezcan, and A. Semercioz, "The Efficacy of Citalopram in the Treatment of Premature Ejaculation: A Placebo-Controlled Study," *International Journal of Impotence Research* 14, no. 6 (December 2002): 502–505.

4: Infertility: Not Just a Woman's Problem

1. C. D. Pavlovich and P. N. Schlegel, "Cost-Effectiveness of Treatment for Male Infertility," *Assisted Reproduction Reviews* 8, no. 1 (1998): 40–46.

2. M. Hansen, J. J. Kurinczuk, C. Bower, and S. Webb, "The Risk of Major Birth Defects After Intracytoplasmic Sperm Injection and *in Vitro* Fertilization," *The New England Journal of Medicine* 346 (March 7, 2002): 725–730.

3. F. Y. Kim and M. Goldstein, "Antibacterial Skin Preparation Decreases the Incidence of False-Positive Semen Culture Results," *The Journal of Urology* 161 (1999): 819–821.

4. C. Rolf, S. Kenkel, and E. Nieschlag, "Age-Related Disease Pattern in Infertile Men: Increasing Incidence of Infections in Older Patients," *Andrologia* 34 (2002): 209–217.

5. J. I. Gorelick and M. Goldstein, "Loss of Fertility in Men with Varicocele," *Fertility and Sterility* 59, no. 3 (1993): 613–616.

6. H. Fisch, G. Hyun, and T. W. Hensle, "Testicular Growth and Gonadotrophin Response Associated with Varicocele Repair in Adolescent Males," *BJU International* 91, no. 1 (January 2003): 75–78.

7. World Health Organization, "A Double-Blind Trial of Clomiphene Citrate for the Treatment of Idiopathic Male Infertility," *International Journal of Andrology* 15, vol. 4 (August 1992): 299–307.

5: Finding Sperm When a Man Is "Sterile"

1. 2001 Assisted Reproductive Technology Success Rates. U.S. Department of Health and Human Services, Centers for Disease Control. 2003. p. 11.
2. Web site of the American Society for Reproductive Medicine, www.asrm.org/Patients/faqs.html#Q6, accessed January 16, 2004.
3. Reported in L. R. Schover and A. J. Thomas, *Overcoming Male Infertility* (New York: John Wiley & Sons, 2000), p. 158.

6: Slowing the Biological Clock: A Guide to Sexual Health

1. E. A. Saltzman, A. T. Guay, and J. Jacobson, "Improvement in Erectile Function in Men with Organic Erectile Dysfunction by Correction of Elevated Cholesterol Levels: A Clinical Observation," *The Journal of Urology* 172, no. 1 (July 2004): 255–258.
2. J. E. Joy, S. J. Watson, and J. A. Benson (eds.), *Marijuana and Medicine: Assessing the Science Base* (Washington, D.C.: National Academy Press, 1999), p. 104.

Acknowledgments

A book like this one requires the help of many people. Here are just a few who made it possible and whom I thank immensely: Dr. Larry Lipshultz and Dr. Carl Olsson are the people who inspired me to become a urologist specializing in male reproductive health. Columbia University is a special place with special people, including the faculty and staff in the Department of Urology, the nurses and staff at the Allen Pavilion, and the medical students who inspire me every day. As for the patients whom I have treated: I consider it an honor that you allowed me to be your doctor and I thank you for continually teaching me about the importance of family. I also want to thank my good friend and statistician Gary Liberson for his help with the many statistics in this book. Last, but not least, are the special people in the publishing industry: Bruce Nichols and Leslie Meredith at Free Press saw something that was possible and really made it happen; and Gail Ross, my agent, whom I admire for her insights, intellect, and ability to lead by example. Thank you all!

Index

Index

About the Authors

Harry Fisch, M.D., is Director of the Male Reproductive Center at Columbia University Medical Center of New York Presbyterian Hospital, in New York City. He is also professor of clinical urology at Columbia University, where he was recently named Urology Teacher of the Year. He is an American Board of Urology Diplomate and a Fellow of the American College of Surgeons. For more than fifteen years, Dr. Fisch has focused his research and practice on male infertility and reproduction, publishing and lecturing widely. In his private practice in Manhattan, Dr. Fisch has successfully treated thousands of men with fertility problems. He is widely recognized as an expert in his field, having been quoted in publications such as *The New York Times* and *The Economist,* and appearing on shows such as *The Today Show* and the CBS evening news.

Stephen Braun is an award-winning medical writer and producer. He is the author of a number of articles in such publications as *Science* and *The Boston Globe,* as well as three books: *The Science and Lore of Alcohol and Caffeine; The Science of Happiness: Unlocking the Mysteries of Mood;* and *The Peace of Mind Prescription.*